DATE DUE FOR RETURN

14 OCT 1993 04PM

Doing
Feminist
Research

Also edited by Helen Roberts

Women, Health and Reproduction

Doing
Feminist
Research

Edited by
Helen Roberts

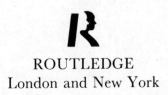

ROUTLEDGE
London and New York

First published in 1981
by Routledge & Kegan Paul plc

Reprinted 1982, 1984, 1986, 1988

Reprinted 1990 by Routledge
11 New Fetter Lane, London EC4P 4EE
29th West 35th Street, New York NY 10001
Reprinted 1990

Set in IBM Baskerville 11 on 12pt by
Hope Services (Abingdon) Ltd
and printed in Great Britain by
Redwood Burn Ltd, Trowbridge, Wiltshire

British Library Cataloguing in Publication Data
Doing feminist research
1. Women
I. Roberts, Helen
305.4   HQ1206   80–42164
ISBN 0–415–02547–8

Contents

v

Acknowledgments

Various people have given practical and intellectual help in the production of this book, particularly women from the Sexual Divisions Study Group and the Women's Caucus of the British Sociological Association. William Outhwaite gave helpful advice on the translation of Christine Delphy's chapter and Irene Booth, Joyce Pates, Maureen Pollard and Lorna Todd helped with the typescript.

Notes on contributors

Lynne Chisholm is a sociologist, currently lecturing in sociology and anthropology at the University of Maryland, West Germany. Her publications include exploration of links between sex, marital status and suicide, and the career development of single women. She is currently hoping to develop a project investigating processes of occupational choice for girls/women in West Germany and the United Kingdom.

Christine Delphy was born in Paris in 1941 and was educated at the Sorbonne, the University of Chicago and the University of California at Berkeley. She is a full-time research fellow in sociology with the Centre Nationale de la Recherche Scientifique, and is an editor of the journal *Questions Feministes*. She has been a participant in the radical feminist current since the beginning of the French women's liberation movement, and is presently working on the political economy of the family.

Catriona Llewellyn was Research Officer in the Social Mobility Group at Nuffield College, Oxford from 1972 to 1976. She was subsequently a research executive with the Opinion Research Centre and is currently Senior Research Officer with the Training Services Division, Manpower Services Commission. She conducted her research into women in banks while in Oxford. More recently she has been involved in identifying training initiatives for women as part of a UK report — *Training for Equality* — prepared by the MSC for the European Centre for the Development of Vocational Training.

David Morgan has taught in the Department of Sociology at Manchester University since 1964. He is author of *Social Theory and the Family* (Routledge & Kegan Paul, 1975) and various other papers on the sociology of the family. This, together with the sociology of literature, remains a chief interest but he would like to explore further some themes in the study of men and masculinity.

Ann Oakley is currently Honorary Research Officer, Bedford College, University of London, and Wellcome Research Fellow, National Perinatal Epidemiology Unit, Churchill Hospital, Oxford, working on the history of antenatal care in Britain. She is the author of *Becoming a Mother* (Martin Robertson, 1979), *Women Confined: Towards a Sociology of Childbirth* (Martin Robertson, 1980), and *The Sociology of Housework* (Martin Robertson, 1974).

Joyce J. M. Pettigrew currently lectures at Queen's University, Belfast, and is undertaking research in the rural areas of the Punjab on infant illness and death during weaning. She was a member of a Sikh family for seven years and is author of *Robber Noblemen* (Routledge & Kegan Paul, 1975) and various articles. She graduated with a PhD from Manchester where she was a pupil of Max Gluckman.

Helen Roberts is Senior Researcher at Ilkley College where she is currently working on the reception and resettlement of Vietnamese refugees. Her main research interest is in the health of women and she has done work on the menopause and on contraception.

Dale Spender is an Australian who lives in London. She is editor of *Women's Studies International Quarterly* and editor and author of feminist books which are concerned with male control of the construction of knowledge, including *Man Made Language* (Routledge & Kegan Paul, 1980).

Diana Woodward took a BA in Social Science at Leicester University, and a PhD at Cambridge on the situation of women in male-dominated disciplines. From 1973 to 1976 she worked on a study of 1960 graduates at Sheffield University, and since 1976 has been Senior Lecturer in Sociology at Sheffield City Polytechnic. She has been an active member of the Committee for the Equality of the Sexes of the British Sociological Association, was a member of the BSA Executive, and has been involved in the activities of the Women's Caucus and the NATFHE Women's Group at the Polytechnic.

Ten Years On

Helen Roberts

Ten years have passed since preparation was started on the collection of essays which appear in *Doing Feminist Research*. In the normal course of events, one might have expected a completely new edition after a decade. But it is clear that whatever the shortcomings of the book there is a sense in which, as the first British book in this area, it has become something of a classic. If I were the writer, rather than the editor of this collection, British modesty and reserve would have prevented me from making this point, but I am glad to say that it is true, and the book has been widely cited and well used. It was therefore felt by the publishers, by me, and by those of the authors I spoke to that it was worth keeping the collection in print in its present form. This supplementary introduction, one decade on, reviews the reception of the collection, looks at some aspects of its impact, and draws attention to continuing methodological problems for those practising feminist research in the social sciences.

Doing feminist research and the gatekeepers

Dale Spender, in her chapter in this book, examines four issues around 'gatekeeping' in the academic community.

These are the significance of publishing, and attitudes towards it, the role played by publications in shaping a discipline, the criteria used for determining scholarly excellence, and the problem of male domination in publishing. It is perhaps worth exploring some of these issues in relation to *Doing Feminist Research*.

In 1978, I was teaching a postgraduate course in research methodology at the University of Bradford and found the collection of essays edited by Colin Bell and Howard Newby (Bell and Newby, 1977), in which researchers reflected on their personal experience of social research, useful, lively, and a real antidote to some of the dry methods textbooks I was recommending. A gap in this collection was that there was no mention of feminism, nor were there any contributions from women. I wrote to the publisher's editor at Allen and Unwin with a proposal for the book, which was to become *Doing Feminist Research*. He replied:

> At the time *Doing Sociological Research* was planned, we were mainly looking for major research projects from which important and seminal accounts had been published in book form. . . . I do not think that the necessity or otherwise of a feminist methodological contribution ever really occurred to us. We were not intending the book to be comprehensive, or to cover all styles or modes of research. So I would not accept what you say about the significance of an absence of female research in the Bell and Newby book . . . All that being said, and with the omission (if not the admission of it) made, then we are left with a rather small and specifically feminist market for the kind of book you have in mind. . . .

The book was taken on by Philippa Brewster, a feminist editor at Routledge, who has since founded a successful feminist imprint, Pandora. The book did well, but the Allen and Unwin editor may have been correct about the 'specifically feminist market', though now it is by no means small. Certainly one is more likely to find *Doing Feminist Research* cited in the work of feminists and fellow travellers than in mainstream sociology texts, though one of the essays, that by Ann Oakley, has been the focus of debate in a mainstream journal (Malseed, 1987; Oakley, 1987).

Doing Feminist Research is more likely to appear on reading lists for Women's Studies courses than for research methods courses. A recent review of methods textbooks puts the Bell and Newby collection in the top ten for both sociology degrees and combined courses, while *Doing Feminist Research* does not appear at all (Payne *et. al.*, 1989). The authors comment 'It is . . . interesting to note . . . the relative absence of sources in the list on feminist research and interpersonal skills such as interviewing' (p. 266). The article makes clear that in terms of qualitative research, the Chicago school continues to dominate and the universes suitable for study are schools, deviant sub-cultures, and occupations. What makes this so depressing for those of us working within a feminist tradition is that, as the authors point out: 'For the professional sociologist, "research" is not a separate, specialist domain, but rather a part of the *practice* of sociology. In contrast, the teaching of Methods has for a long time continued to treat research as if it were quite independent of other aspects of the discipline' (p. 262).

How was the book received by reviewers? On the whole, it was treated kindly in both the sociological and the feminist literature. *Doing Feminist Research* explicitly drew on some of the tradition (if that is not too pretentious a word for something so new) of 'telling it like it is' accounts of sociological research (Bell and Encel, 1979; Bell and Newby, 1977). One difference was that the essays in *Doing Feminist Research* were not to be used as a vehicle for settling old scores, sniping, or continuing the rather machismo sport of intellectual cut and thrust, amusing though those aspects of the earlier collections had sometimes been. It was gratifying, therefore, to read in Bell's (1981) review: '. . . it gives me great sexist pleasure to report that it is far less gossipy than other similar collections – that will, I suspect, particularly disappoint male readers' (p. 323). There was, I believe, a feeling among some readers that a feminist approach would be a cosy sort of women's magazine didacticism, the intellectual equivalent of a fireside chat. Notwithstanding the discussion of objectivity in the first chapter, there was some alarm concerning what might be interpreted as a lack of scientific rigour and objectivity. Wakeford (1982, p. 144), who wrote a favourable review of the book for *Sociology* and who was generally sympathetic to the feminist approach outlined in the collection, cautioned: 'If we reject the canons of academic and scientific rationality we must ask what standards *are* to be employed for research practice . . .'

It seemed to me then, as it does now, that good feminist research, rather than rejecting academic and scientific rationality, is proposing that we critically re-examine socially constructed notions of just what it is that constitutes scholarship and rationality. What good feminist scholarship has done, far from jettisoning 'the canons of academic and scientific rationality', is to begin applying them more widely and more radically and to use them to question principles and assumptions whose justification and explanation had a great deal to do with gender divisions and very little to do with the pursuit of knowledge. How rational is it, for instance, in a sociology in which social class plays such a central part, to rely on a social classification scheme in which married women are classified according to the occupation of a husband on whom they may or may not depend?

Social classification is a fundamental methodological problem and two chapters in the present volume are devoted to a discussion of this topic. Christine Delphy's elegant essay 'Women in stratification studies' and Catriona Llewellyn's 'Occupational mobility and the use of the comparative method' were early contributions to the women and social class debate, although by no means the first. Early feminist critiques of the social classification of women can be found in the work of Acker (1973) and Haug (1973) and there has been a considerable body of largely theoretical literature on the social classification of women in the decade since *Doing Feminist Research* was produced.

Objections to the current conventional classification range from the ideological – that it is offensive to many that married women should be classified according to the occupation of a husband on whom they may or may not be dependent – to the straightforwardly logical: that to classify a woman in terms of her own occupation until the day she marries, but from then on to classify her in terms of the occupation of her husband (whether or not she is in paid work) is inconsistent. There is good evidence (Graham, 1984; Land, 1980) that the resources of the household are not equally shared, which weakens the case that the household is the appropriate unit of stratification (and the occupation of the male 'head of household' most useful for this purpose).

Among objections to the classification of women using existing scales are the inability of these to distinguish sufficiently finely between women's occupations, problems concerning the manual/non-manual divide, and the concentration of a very large number of women in a very small number of occupations. Current conventions of classification do not distinguish between full and part-time workers, and for those women whose labour is in the home and unwaged, there is no classification scheme at all. While there has been a good deal of theoretical work, and critiques, counter-critiques, and replies (*Sociology* volume 17 no. 4, volume 18 nos. 2 and 4), rather less has been achieved at a practical level, though a number of alternatives have been proposed (Martin and Roberts, 1984; Dale *et. al.*, 1985; Barker and Roberts, 1986). Delphy's chapter in this collection argues that problems of social class classification should not be viewed simply as methodological errors or ideological biases. In other words, the present problem of the classification of women for social class purposes does not simply represent a superficial flaw.

This is made amply clear in Heidi Mirza's (1985) work investigating the ways in which gender and race effect educational outcomes for young black women. She points out how inappropriate it is to classify West Indian children by their fathers' occupation in families which are frequently headed by females. As Mirza points out, this convention is based on an ethnocentric assumption concerning the nature of family structure and the distributution of resources within the family. Mirza's Emperor and Clothes observation underlines the gap between data, theory, and classifications.

In recent years, there have been substantial criticisms of major studies which have failed to look at women in terms of social class, and feminists in particular have argued that large-scale funding of studies which fail to take women into account is not money well spent. Neither the Oxford Mobility Group, which studied occupational mobility in England and Wales, nor the Scottish Occupational Survey included females in their samples, although the Scottish study did collect information on wives. But as the authors of the latter study themselves point out (Payne *et. al.*, 1981), the wives of a random sample of men are not a random sample of women. They exclude single, widowed, divorced, and separated women, and their selection is dependent upon the selection of their partners. Responses to the feminist critique have borne a marked similarity to Billy Bunter's cry: 'I didn't take that cake. And it wasn't a very nice cake anyway'. But ironically enough, as Sarah Delamont (1989) points out, the emergence of one of the main proponents, John Goldthorpe, into the debate *'itself* gives greater credence to the criticisms of stratification theory as sexist (p. 335).'

Goldthorpe writes:

> Taken at face value, such [feminist] critiques may be thought cogent. However, they appear somewhat less impressive once more attention is given to their alleged target. For, on closer examination of the matter, it becomes clear that the conventional view which they seek to oppose occurs in more than one version. While it is true that most stratification theorists *have* treated the family as the unit of stratification, and have been crucially dependent on the location of the family head within the occupational division of labour, what needs also to be recognised is that this view has been arrived at through different and . . . sharply contrasting theoretical routes' (Goldthorpe, 1983, pp. 465–6).

Stanworth (1984), replying to Goldthorpe, argues that the conventional approach which he defends both obscures the extent to which the class experience of wives differs from that of husbands, and ignores the extent to which the inequalities that divide women and men are themselves the outcome of the operation of the class system.

A useful classification of women is not, of course, merely a question of ideological niceties, though it may be noted that no man, whether in or out of employment, is classified according to the occupation of the woman to whom he is attached by marriage. Attempts that have been made so far to integrate women into existing categorisations are derived from assumptions about work (that it is paid, full-time, and continuous), which may work reasonably well for most men, but not for most women.

Any serious attempt to look at the social classification of women needs to begin from the realities of women's lives rather than attempting to awkwardly fit them into pre-existing categories. A classification of women should derive from the sorts of lives women lead, and not from categories derived from the realities of the lives of working men. This issue remains unresolved.

The issue of social class, since it is so central to mainstream sociology, serves as a good illustration of a fundamental point raised by Margaret Stacey in her review of *Doing Feminist Research*. She noted: 'The papers . . . demonstrate . . . how far we still have to go before we achieve a sociology, not only a methodology, which can see beyond the confines of the society in which it is embedded' (Stacey, 1981). Certainly there has been an enormous growth in the women's studies area over the last ten years and a collection of women's studies books which might have taken up a couple of shelves a decade ago now require a bookshop. But how far is mainstream sociology affected? Feminist scholarship has still to make a major impact in the social sciences. It is still an outsider saying 'yes, but' to the conventional wisdoms, rather than the source of an enhanced perspective which takes gender into account as a matter of course. If feminist scholarship is causing alarm, that may be because it is winning some influence. But it hasn't yet by any means won the war.

The aims of *Doing Feminist Research* are relatively modest. The book simply raises a number of problematic methodo-logical issues for those doing empirical studies. The rather grand title was a play on the title of Bell and Newby's *Doing Sociological Research* rather than an attempt to provide a blueprint for feminist research. It is hardly surprising that in their review of methods textbooks, referred to above, Payne *et.*

al. bracket together feminist research with interpersonal skills. Feminist research is frequently equated with qualitative research, which is, I believe, mistaken. *Doing Feminist Research* like much subsequent work on feminist research (Stanley and Wise, 1983; Bell and Roberts, 1984; Harding 1987; Smith 1988) is largely concerned with theoretical and qualitative issues. If I were getting together a similar collection now, I would have more feminist work using quantitative techniques.

The quantitative/qualitative divide has recently been addressed by Ann Oakley who argues that:

> Although feminist research practice requires a critical stance towards existing methodology . . . at the same time, it has to be recognised that the universe of askable research questions is constrained by the methods allowed. To ban any quantitative (social) science therefore results in a restriction to certain kinds of questions only; this restriction may very well be counter to the same epistemological goal a code of feminist research practice is designed to promote (Oakley, 1990).

This collection does not offer an answer to the question 'What is feminist research?' nor is it intended to. To offer a knitting pattern approach would be to deny the diversity and creativity of research, and worse, could replace prescriptions of what is sociologically or scientifically 'right' with prescriptions of what is, from a feminist point of view, 'right on'. I hope that this collection will continue to provide a starting point for researchers who are themselves doing feminist research.

Helen Roberts
Glasgow 1989

References

Acker, J. (1973) 'Women and stratification: a case of intellectual sexism', *American Journal of Sociology* vol. 78, pp. 936–45.

Barker, R. and Roberts, H. (1986) 'A social classification scheme for women', working paper no. 46, Social Statistics Research Unit, City University, London.

Bell, C. (1981) 'A question of gender', *New Society* 21 May, vol. 56, no. 966, p. 323.

Bell, C. and Encel, S. (1979) *Inside the Whale*, Pergamon, Australia.

Bell, C. and Newby, H. (eds.) (1977) *Doing Sociological Research*, Allen and Unwin, London.

Bell, C. and Roberts, H. (1984) *Social Researching, Politics, Problems and Practice*, Routledge and Kegan Paul, London.

Dale, A., Gilbert, G.N., and Arber, S. (1985) 'Integrating women into class theory', *Sociology* vol. 19, pp. 384–409.

Delamont, S. (1989) 'Research note: citation and social mobility research: self defeating behaviour?' *Sociological Review* pp. 332–37.

Goldthorpe, J. (1983) 'Women and class analysis,' *Sociology* vol. 17, pp. 465–88.

Goldthorpe, J. (1984) 'Women and class analysis: a reply to the replies', *Sociology* vol. 18, pp. 491–9.

Graham, H. (1984) *Women, Health and the Family*, Wheatsheaf Books, Brighton.

Harding, S. (ed.) (1987) *Feminism and Methodology*, Open University Press, Milton Keynes.

Haug, M. (1973) 'Social class measurement and women's occupational roles', *Social Forces* vol. 52, pp. 86–98.

Land, H. (1980) 'The family wage', *Feminist Review* no. 6, pp. 55–78.

Malseed, J. (1987) 'Straw men: a note on Ann Oakley's treatment of textbook prescriptions for interviewing', *Sociology* vol. 21, no. 4, pp. 629–31.

Martin, J. and Roberts, C. (1984) *Women and Employment: A Lifetime Perspective*, HMSO, London.

Mirza, H. (1985) 'Distortions of social reality: a case for reappraising social class schema definitions'. (Paper presented to the Postgraduate Women's Seminar, University of London, Goldsmith's College.)

Oakley, A. (1987) 'Comment on Malseed', *Sociology* vol. 21, no. 4, p. 632.

Oakley, A. (1990) 'Who's afraid of the randomized controlled trial?', Helen Roberts (ed.) *Women's Health Counts* Routledge, London.

Payne, G., Ford, C., and Ulas, M. (1981) 'Occupational change and social mobility in Scotland since the First World War', in M. Gaskin (ed.) *The Political Economy of Tolerable Survival*, Croom Helm, London.

Payne, G., Lyon, E.S., and Anderson, R. (1989) 'Undergraduate sociology: research methods in the public sector curriculum', *Sociology* vol. 23, no. 2, pp. 261–74.

Smith, D. (1988) *The Everyday World as Problematic: A Feminist Sociology*, Open University Press, Milton Keynes.

Stacey, M. (1981) Review of *Doing Feminist Research* in *Network*, Newsletter of the British Sociological Association.

Stanley, L. and Wise, S. (1983) *Breaking Out: Feminist Consciousness and Feminist Research*, Routledge and Kegan Paul, London.

Stanworth, M. (1984) 'Women and class analysis: a reply to Goldthorpe', *Sociology* vol. 18, pp. 159–70.

Wakeford, J. (1982) Review of *Doing Feminist Research* in *Sociology* vol. 16 no. 1 pp. 142–44.

Introduction

Helen Roberts

It must be clear to even the most traditional of male scholars that we can no longer follow Evans Pritchard's advice to 'behave like a gentleman, keep off the women, take quinine daily and play it by ear'.

The aim of this collection of papers is to present a number of accounts of sociological work undertaken by sociologists who have been influenced by feminism, or by the feminist critique of sociology, or both.

Recent works such as Bell and Newby's *Doing Sociological Research* (1977), Bell and Encel's *Inside the Whale* (1978), and Platt's *The Realities of Social Research* (1976) have indicated the very real problems which frequently underlie the polished accounts resulting from completed research. This collection, proceeding on the basis that problems raised in personal accounts of research are themselves of sociological importance, and that such accounts can give the student a lively insight into research often denied by conventional methodology textbooks, examines some of the theoretical, practical, ethical and methodological issues raised by the recognition that social processes are affected by sexual as well as class divisions.

Given the subject matter of sociology and its concern with social structure and social change, given a significant interest in the discipline in the sociology of social movements, and given the resurgence of the women's movement in the late 1960s, an understanding of the importance of sexual divisions in society could not be ignored within the discipline. But much of the work which has appeared on sexual divisions has been very much concerned, in Oakley's terms, with making women 'visible' within sociology. There has been little basic theoretical work, and less still on the ways in which either taking a feminist perspective, or even merely taking account of women in research affects the research process.

The accounts in this collection point to theoretical, methodological, practical and ethical issues raised in projects where the investigator has adopted, or has at least become aware of, a feminist perspective.

The first chapter, which arose from an SSRC workshop on qualitative data, explores some of the background issues in doing a piece of feminist research, and discusses whether the terms feminist or non-sexist methodology are useful ones. The chapter looks at the inadequacy of data bases in this area in formulating research proposals, the organisation of the research team, and the accessibility of research findings.

Ann Oakley's chapter addresses itself to the problems raised for feminist social scientists in adopting the standard criteria of interviewing as laid down in the methods text-books. Oakley discusses the difficulties of finding a way out of the particular problems of interviewing and gives attention to the challenge posed by longtitudinal interviewing practice, and to the issue, prominent in her transition to motherhood study, of the number and kind of questions asked by interviewees of interviewers. She suggests that not only does feminism necessarily contravene the axioms of interviewing as established in the methods textbooks, but that these textbook descriptions of how social scientists should or do obtain their data are based on a masculine view of social reality which is fundamentally at odds with the viewpoints of women as social actors.

Joyce Pettigrew's chapter similarly raises issues which are not addressed by conventional methods textbooks. In her chapter Pettigrew looks back on her own research situation among landowning Sikhs (Jats) during a first fieldwork trip to the Punjab in 1965–7 which resulted in the publication of *Robber Noblemen*. In her very personal account, the author seeks to present and examine the nature of the two most important variables affecting her own fieldwork conditions in the Punjab: that of being a young western woman anthropologist and of being married to a Jat. She discusses both the assets and disadvantages of the position she held in the society studied and raises the difficult issue of whether a woman is in fact suited to gather information in societies whose social organisation is influenced by the notion of purdah, and who is therefore able to gather only a small part of the data she knows to be available. Although the problem of access is raised in other chapters, it is in this chapter that the problems are raised in their most acute form.

Reversing the normal gender distribution in publications of this type, David Morgan's chapter is the only contribution from a male sociologist. In the light of the critique of normal sociological practice coming from the contemporary women's movement, Morgan looks reflexively at his own work and his position as a male sociologist. In his discussion, he assumes that the term 'non-sexist methodology' refers less to the adoption or non-adoption of particular techniques of data collection and analysis and more to the wider matter of the social relations of sociological production. His discussion is illustrated with examples taken from his work: a study of the social and educational backgrounds of Anglican bishops, a participant observation study of a northern factory, and some current work on the 'Bloomsbury' group. In his discussion, Morgan argues first that the central requirement of a non-sexist methodology is that of always taking gender seriously, which is by no means a simple business; second that up to now 'taking gender into account' has usually meant taking women into account. A non-sexist methodology should, in a literal sense, 'bring men back in'; third that most women currently engaged in sociological work do not need to be told the significance of gender; their own experience confirms this. Men on the other hand — in taking gender into account — are going against the grain. Finally he argues that the reason why men must be seen as working against the grain in this respect is the male dominance of universities and other research and teaching institutions. How far, as a result of this, the dominant rationality is a male rationality is a complex question in the sociology of science and the philosophy of science, which Morgan attempts to examine in his chapter.

Studies of the significance of social class are central to British sociology, yet it is frequently argued that it is technically difficult if not impossible to classify women by occupation. Christine Delphy, a French sociologist, analyses the flaws and inadequacies in studies of class which fail to explain the class position of women.

Catriona Llewellyn develops this crucial discussion of women in stratification studies in her description of work carried out while she was employed on a major study of social mobility. Although this study was confined to the male population, Llewellyn and a colleague initiated with very limited resources a small comparative study of men and women in banking using a conventional mobility approach. In her chapter, Llewellyn outlines the findings of this piece of research, and discusses the implications of these for conventional studies of occupational mobility. Although this particular issue is not discussed in Llewellyn's chapter, it is interesting in terms of the research team (if team is the appropriate term in a context which is normally a very rigid hierarchy) to note that as is often the case, the research content and design were already established by the time she was employed, thus raising the general issue of support staff being brought in at a stage where the research programme is already planned.

Following Llewellyn's account, Diana Woodward and Lynne Chisholm discuss the problems which arose from their feminist approach while working on the second national survey of 1960 graduates. A first problem was that of the researchers' presentation of self to the interviewees, and the extent to which they felt they could (relatively accurately) be categorised by respondents in terms of probable life styles, norms and values. For the women interviewed, the researchers represented a role option which many of them had 'chosen' to repudiate, namely pursuing a full-time career. It was also felt that there might be difficulties in establishing rapport between the (childless) interviewers and the women giving accounts of motherhood. A related problem was that of the presentation of research topic to interviewees. The researchers wanted to determine how far the experiences of men and women differed, for example whether similar structural opportunities, norms, values and ideologies had influenced their careers and their performance of family roles, or whether major differences existed which could be explained in terms of social structure, socialisation, differential distribution of power and resources, etc. The researchers thus had to consider carefully how to explain and present the research to the interviewees as a potential conflict existed between the researchers' feminist perspective and the relatively sex-differentiated perspectives of most of the respondents. In their contribution, the authors discuss their recognition of these methodological issues, and the strategies they adopted to deal with them are illustrated with verbatim quotations from the interview transcripts.

A substantial section of the first chapter deals with one aspect of the research process which is frequently omitted — that of the literature forming the intellectual background to the research. The final chapter looks at the other end of the research process — also frequently omitted from discussions of research — and this is the issue of publication. Dale Spender, who edits a feminist journal and a series of feminist academic books, uses her experience as an editor to write an informed polemic on the publication of research findings. Spender looks at the part played by publications in shaping a discipline and suggests that the 'gatekeeping' function of editors is one which should be given serious consideration.

Women form a relatively high proportion of the constituency of researchers: a fact which has not always been reflected in collections of this type. This may of course be partly due to the tendency for women in the research team to be concentrated in the less powerful posts, working as research assistants, data processors or secretaries. It is to be hoped that the high concentration of work by women sociologists in this collection will serve as a reminder of the part women play in carrying out sociological research, while David Morgan's contribution underlines the importance of the feminist critique of sociology to all sociologists.

Helen Roberts, Ilkley, 1980

References

Bell, Colin and Encel, S. (1979), *Inside the Whale*, Pergamon, Australia.

Bell, Colin and Newby, Howard (eds) (1977), *Doing Sociological Research*, Allen & Unwin, London.

Platt, Jennifer (1976), *Realities of Social Research: An Empirical Study of British Sociologists*, University of Sussex Press, London.

1

Women and their doctors:

power and powerlessness in the research process[1]

Helen Roberts

This chapter, although drawing on a particular research project, attempts to raise in a preliminary way issues which are developed in more detail in subsequent chapters, and to look at general problems concerning the development of particular ways of doing research which can be related to a wider feminist perspective in sociology.

In recent years some sociologists (mostly feminists) have been tackling the problem of the 'invisibility' of women in sociological enquiry. During this time, although some attention has been paid at the level of informal discussion (for instance within the British Sociological Association Womens Caucus) to problematic methodological issues for those working within a feminist framework, little has been written on the subject.

In 1977, Helen Roberts and Michèle Barrett, working together on a sociological analysis of womens' consulting rates at their general practitioner, were asked to contribute to a workshop on qualitative methodology where the organisers suggested that papers should focus on the 'intellectual rather than the practical or "political" problems of qualitative research'. It seemed at the time that it was not only in this particular piece of research that a separation of the intellectual from the practical and the political was problematic, but this

7

research, by adopting a framework in which the women studied were subjects *rather than objects, may have rendered the 'political' problems more evident. In what follows, Helen Roberts looks at some of the issues raised by the use of a feminist perspective in theory and practice as well as in methodological issues.*

Grace: They call me Grace.
Yesterday I went
to the grocery store.
I had filled up
the cart
and was halfway through
the check stand
before I realised
I had shopped for the whole family.
The last child left
two years ago.
I don't know what
got into
me.
I was too embarrassed
to take things back
so I spent the week cooking
casseroles.
I feel like one of those
eternal motion machines
designed for an
obsolete task
that just keeps on
running
I certainly don't want them
back either.
When the
last baby stopped getting
up at
night, I didn't stop . . .
. . . And William never
understood. To him

if you are tired, you sleep.
I have never been able to
penetrate the
simplicity of his logic
which is
after all
the logic
of most of the world. (Griffin, 1975, p.35)[2]

This extract from Susan Griffin's poetry play *Voices* (1975)
serves as an illustration of some of the central concerns in
looking at the consulting rates of middle-aged women at the
doctor's surgery. The first part of the quotation points in a
very acute way to the feelings of some middle-aged women
after their children have left home and they perceive themselves (and are frequently, if implicitly, perceived by others
to be) socially obsolete. The second section, which refers to

'the logic
of most of the world'

provides a starting point for some of the methodological issues
I should like to discuss.

Our research on women and their doctors was begun in the
light of the well documented fact that women have higher
consultation rates with their GPs than do men, that middle-
aged women have a particularly high discrepancy with men in
this respect once consultations for childbirth and contraception in the younger age group of women are taken into account,[3] and from the widely held view that a good deal of the
complaints of high consulters in this age group are seen as
'psychosomatic' in origin. We held the view that the label
'psychosomatic' as applied to the complaints presented by
certain groups of women was less apposite than the parallel
term 'sociosomatic'[4] since the latter acknowledged the social
basis of such psychological phenomena. We held that the social
and economic structure of modern industrial society systematically causes women to be disadvantaged educationally,
occupationally, and in other ways. This disadvantaged position, as Friedan (1973) and others have suggested, may have

as its result vague feelings of dissatisfaction and minor worries and complaints. We wanted to explore the possibility that women in this position, particularly women with little interest outside their families (and therefore most vulnerable at middle age as their children leave home) use their doctor as a source of attention and sympathy as well as a source of compensation for the frustrations and inadequacies of their daily lives. (In fact, we found that their visits to the doctor were more than this, and that the doctor played a more active part in reconciling women to their traditionally prescribed role.)

Preliminary research we had done indicated that an analysis of ideological factors in general practice consultations was essential, and we were inevitably led in formulating our work into a discussion of the general practitioner's attitudes towards his or her patients. These attitudes were, we found, particularly relevant in relation to the gender of patients, which the doctor perceived as an important influence in determining their priorities in life. We also found that it would be necessary to look at the patient's attitudes towards her doctor, and the congruence between these attitudes, those of the doctor, and those of ancillary staff and specialists. Hence, as well as approaching the study in such a way as to secure qualitative and quantitative data, we wanted to approach it from the doctor's view as well as from the patient's. It seemed to us at the stage when we were setting up the research, that the doctor's perception of a patient's sex (and what he or she takes to be the consequences of it) would affect diagnosis and treatment in much the same way as his or her perception of other socially significant variables such as class and occupation. This perception and its consequences, we hypothesised, would vary in relation to the doctor's age, sex and medical training as well as in relation to his or her social class background and practice experience.

We hypothesised that women patients' perception and use of medical services would be influenced by age, employment, position in the family life cycle and so on. For these reasons, we chose to work within a sample which, at the same time as supplying us with the qualitative data, would allow us to compare consulting behaviour in terms of a range of variables. Eight study practices were used, constituted in the following manner: 4 surburban, 2 inner city, 2 rural. The sample was weighted towards surburban residential areas because of the high proportion of full-time housewives there. We worked with both male and female doctors and covered such variables as age, social class background, training and single-handed and group practices in the sample. While the sample of practices was too small to allow for a statistically significant comparison on the basis of these variables, we felt at least that we could guard against such variables potentially vitiating our research. ('Ah, but you haven't looked at women/young/old/group/ health centre/single-handed doctors.')

Within each of the practices a sample of thirty women was selected on the following basis to be studied in detail:

(a)   From the age/sex register, a list of women born between 1921 and 1931 was compiled.
(b)   For these women records were consulted and the frequency of consultations over the past five years noted.
(c)   From these rates, a list was drawn up of the fifteen highest and fifteen lowest consulters in a given practice, and these women constituted the sample for the practice. These women were then approached by letter for an interview, and, with their permission, their records and any correspondence passing between the GP and specialists, analysed in more detail.

Each of the respondents took part in a long semi-structured interview in her own home conducted by one of the two investigators. In response to a request from the SSRC who funded the research, two samples of male patients were also interviewed, an issue which will be discussed below.

Although an interview schedule was used, this provided only the basis for the questions to be asked. The interview included basic demographic information, the woman's working history, her health history over the past year and the past five years, her attitudes towards her health and towards her doctor, and her marital history. These interviews lasted anything from three-quarters of an hour in the case of some low consulters to several hours for some of the high consulters. The length of the interview frequently indicated the degree of isolation of the respondent, but also indicated in many cases a very real interest in the research similar to that described by Oakley below.

In addition to this, at least one doctor from each of the practices involved was interviewed. Naturally, one would like to see some evidence that the attitudes and ideological stances expressed by doctors during an interview are consistent with their behaviour during the consultation. One way of approaching this problem would have been to use validation procedures based on actual or simulated consultations, but this was rejected at an early stage for technical and ethical reasons. Since a certain amount of time was spent in each practice, however, giving opportunities for conversation with the doctor as well as the 'interview', and since both patients and doctors were interviewed, the problem of validation was not such an important issue as was originally envisaged.

An additional source of validation, although of a rather more indirect kind, is through a content analysis of professional literature and medical journals dealing with illness among middle-aged women. This analysis served to supplement the discussion of the ideological aspects of the relationship between doctor and patients.

Access to data was less of a problem than might have been supposed. Some of the practices were obtained through the Royal College of General Practitioners Working Party on the Social Components of Disease; others we approached directly. A high response rate was obtained from patients, particularly the high consulters, and this may well be due to the original letter requesting an interview normally coming from the patient's doctor; an indication of the influence of the GP. Before deciding to conduct the research in this way, the possibility of recycling existing data was explored, and of the data resources available, the General Household Survey proved the most relevant. However, no information could be obtained from this survey about the woman's *general* health, and second, of course, the use of this type of survey would have precluded any in depth interviewing on our part. Although some relevant references may be made from the material provided by the survey, the questions asked were not sufficiently specific to our needs for this to be an appropriate way of obtaining data. In addition, since the survey is based on social class position in terms of the husband's occupation, a question raised again below, it poses particular problems in dealing with our hypotheses. The possibility of a large-scale prospective survey was also considered but it was felt that this would be inappropriate given that the qualitative character of the proposed interviewing demanded in our opinion that only the two named investigators carry it out.

The objective of the research, begun in September 1976, was to establish a category of illness, and of demand for medical attention, which would properly be defined as 'sociosomatic'. The concept of psychosomatic illness is known to the general public, has found currency in women's magazines, and is used as a basis for diagnosis and treatment by the medical profession. It was felt, in beginning this research, that the well-documented higher consulting rates at their general practitioner for women,[5,6] and the high incidence among women of 'psychosomatic' complaints and associated disorders could profitably be viewed from a sociological perspective. In doing so, and in setting up the project, it was argued that:

(a) Women are systematically disadvantaged by educational and occupational structures, and are encouraged to see their social role as synonymous with their familial roles as wife and mother; as a consequence of this, the 'dual career' woman often suffers stressful role conflict, and the housewife (particularly at the point of her family cycle at which the children leave home) is vulnerable to feelings of social uselessness, frustration and dissatisfaction. One of the aims of the study was to see how far this distress, so often seen as a manifestation of individual inadequacy, could be viewed in terms of a social structural origin.
(b) Illness of various kinds, and especially the consequent demand for, and gratification obtained by attention from the medical profession, is seen by certain groups of women as a source of compensation for the inadequacies of their daily lives. In this respect, medical attention is parallel to the support traditionally received by women from religious institutions.
(c) The groups of women to whom this hypothesis most directly relates will be sociologically distinct from other groups

of women. Those with no employment outside the home, recent experience of children leaving home, feelings of dissatisfaction with their work, and a lower level of educational and occupational status before marriage are likely to be the most frequent consulters.

(d) The ideological function of the consultation between such a woman and her general practitioner is normally to help her adjust to the limitations of her structurally determined role, rather than to question these limitations. In this respect, the institution of medicine legitimates and endorses the *status quo,* and therefore acts as an agency of disguised social control.

The first point made above relating to social structure has been well documented in recent sociological literature. In this context, Oakley's *Sociology of Housework* (1974) has been an important work, showing as it does in its introductory discussion the way in which sociology itself has traditionally operated within a patriarchal paradigm, and aspects of this will be raised in the discussion below.

An initial problem for those attempting to employ feminist insights concerns accusations of bias and triviality, both of which are rightly seen as being of methodological concern. It was therefore of no real surprise to the investigators to find that the research was subject to at least two streams of criticism. Both of these raised issues concerning 'gatekeeping' and the construction of knowledge discussed in more detail in Dale Spender's chapter.

The first type of criticism was along the lines of: 'SSRC funds another piece of research telling us what we have always known. Any doctor can tell you' (though none in fact did, in this context) 'why middle-aged women spend so much time at the surgery. It's all common sense. When will sociologists do something worthwhile for a change.' Predictably enough, this type of criticism came from some medical practitioners with whom we discussed the research and from certain sections of the medical press.

Rather more interesting was a criticism the research received from within sociology. 'Work had already been done in this area, we were feminists and therefore certainly biased if not worse. Did we not know the scholarly work which documented so well the areas we were trying to examine?' It would be outside the scope of this chapter to respond in a detailed way to these criticisms, but both of them raise an issue which *is* within the scope of the present chapter, and this is the question of bias.

Becker points out that the problem of bias is not merely a problem of technical difficulties to be overcome by stricter and more rigorous methods of research, and suggests that 'The sociologist provokes the charge of bias whenever he says something that denies the legitimacy of the hierarchy of credibility' (Becker, 1971, p.13).

As feminists and as sociologists we challenge the hierarchy of credibility at two levels. We begin by identifying sexism as an ideology, in the sense that it generalises from the experience of one section of society, men, to create an explanation of the experience of both men and women, of the organisation of society as a whole, and of the power relations within it. Such an ideology both denies the experience and objective situation of women, and justifies the distribution of advantages which arises from a sexual division, which division it both ignores and conceals. The ideology is pervasive and largely unarticulated, but it is expressed within sociology by methodologies which ignore sexual divisions and do not 'see' the experience or situation of women. The symptoms of this are familiar, such as the assumption that statements about social class can be made on the basis of male occupations, and that generalisations can be made about all participants from an all-male sample. To those whose methodology is suffused with sexism in this way, a sample composed entirely of men is seen as unproblematical, while one composed entirely of women may be seen as odd, inadequate, or perverse.

Feminism is in the first place an attempt to insist upon the experience and very existence of women. To this extent it is most importantly a feature of an ideological conflict, and does not of itself attempt an 'un-biased' or 'value-free' methodology. Rather by creating a dialectic at the ideological level, it creates the conditions in which a non-sexist methodology might be approached, or at least imagined. Becker, among others, has argued cogently that such value freedom or objectivity is not possible and that 'we cannot avoid taking sides, for reasons firmly based in social structure' (Becker, 1971, p.213). To talk of a feminist methodology is clearly political, controversial and implies personal and/or political sympathies on the part of the researcher which inform but do not constitute the sociological approach. Arlene Daniels (1975), in advocating a feminist perspective, refers to Dorothy Smith (1974), who, she says (p.346),

> underscores the basic limitations of a sociological discipline where women's place is subordinate, ignored, invisible. Women appear only as they are relevant to a world governed by male principles and interests. To the extent that women sociologists accept that perspective, they are alienated from their own personal experience. They speak a language, use theories, and select methods in which they are excluded or ignored.

Feminists, in stressing the need for a reflexive sociology in which the sociologist takes her own experiences seriously and incorporates them into her work, expose themselves to challenges of a lack of objectivity from those of their male colleagues whose sociological insight does not enable them to see that their own work is affected in a similar way by *their* experiences and their view of the world as men. Indeed, as Millman and Kanter suggest, most of the models which dominate sociology focus upon traditionally masculine concerns and male settings.

Some of these problems are not seen as issues by feminists alone. Becker (1971) writes of the constructive use of personal experience in formulating hypotheses and reflexive sociology can hardly be seen as an exclusively feminist concern. Those sociologists who also happen to be feminists (or some might prefer to say those feminists who also happen to be sociologists) are no less professional sociologists than their colleagues and their problems of working in a rigorous manner are no less acute. Indeed, the problems of *not* ignoring a feminist perspective in theory and practice as well as in methodology undoubtedly cause difficulties in the research process. If then, as feminists, we are not giving credence to an established status order, we may open ourselves to criticism both from the profession which we are studying and the profession within which we ourselves practice. On the other hand, we may as feminists allow ourselves to criticise as biased those sociologists who continue to produce work which is sexist in its theories, its methodology, its practice and its application, and who appear unaware of the significance of sexual divisions in society. Counter accusations of bias are not very productive, however, without an analysis of the production and mainten-ance of status order from which the bias is derived, and its associated ideology; a task addressed by the present collection.

One of the ways in which this status order is produced and maintained is through the literature which provides the body of knowledge in an area. This is discussed in greater detail in Spender's chapter, but it is important to note here that a step which is frequently omitted from descriptions of the research process is that of providing a background to the framework within which a piece of research is conceived and developed. Providing such a framework makes explicit the paradigms within which the research is set, and certainly in the mid-1970s when we were preparing our research proposal, the lack of serious attention to sexual divisions in the available material was quite alarming. An examination of this work, however, not only enabled us to formulate more clearly the problem we were examining, but also gave us some indication of the way in which it would be most useful to work (and perhaps more importantly, ways of going about one's work which would not be useful to us).

In turning to the work in the area in question, we noted first a growing body of literature in which medical institutions were conceptualised in social terms. By this, I refer to work based on the simple assumption that social factors operate not only in the use made of medical services, but also in the aetio-logy of disease. This assumption is therefore the fundamental one upon which any explanatory sociology of medicine is based. A notable contribution towards this perspective was made in the volume edited by Dreitzel (1971) in which Katz notes that: 'Chronic low-grade dissatisfaction with their status in life was particularly true of this high illness group of workers' (p.6). Attempts to look at the social causes or func-tions of disease are, however, comparatively rare in the litera-ture. It could well be argued that much sociological literature on medical institutions has been too heavily influenced by the descriptive epidemiological perspective used by the medical profession itself. Hence, although it may be true that the sociology of medicine should be aiming at an explanatory account of differential use of the institutions of medicine, in practice, the literature frequently falls short of this and relies upon descriptive documentation of the social factors at work in any given medical situation.

Notwithstanding the fact that in many cases the sociology of medicine has too readily accepted an epidemiological or descriptive approach, the literature in this area in recent years has shown an increasing awareness of the social factors associated with illness. One consequence of this has been the professional connections established between medicine and social work. Hence Anthony Clare (1976) argues that the social services and medical services should work in close collaboration, and Ratoff's question: 'More Social Work for General Practice?' (1973) is answered emphatically in the affirmative. Perhaps the most important contribution to this section of the literature from the sociology of medicine has been Brown's (1976) work on social causes of disease which has had consequences for the practice of research within medicine itself as well as within the sociology of medicine.

The second major body of literature contributing to the intellectual background of the project related to the concept of illness behaviour. Although now less popular as a perspective within medical sociology, there can be no doubt that the distinction between illness as a biological or physical state, and illness as a social role, has had a profound influence on the discipline in the past. Research stemming from Parson's (1964) work although not necessarily based on Parsonian principles, has been extensive.

Allied to the concept of illness behaviour are studies of 'proneness' to consult a doctor for a given complaint. One such study of particular interest here was that of Wadsworth and his associates who reported that 'persons complaining of headaches were significantly more likely to have gone to the doctor if they were retired . . . or housewives . . . or unemployed' (1971, p.55). Hence it may be argued that certain processes of selection operate in the sequence of events leading to consultation with a general practitioner. In this study, the concept of 'illness behaviour' was used in a flexible way to consider why certain sections of the female population should seek medical attention to a greater degree than others. As suggested above in the findings of Wadsworth *et al.*, it was thought useful to attempt to explore the possibility that women who are tied to the home have more to gain and less to lose by taking refuge in illness behaviour of various kinds.

The third major theme from the existing literature which informed the background to the study concerned the function of medicine as an institution of social control. Undoubtedly the most incisive contribution to this debate has been that made by Zola (1972) in which he argues that the medical profession has taken over an increasingly large area of social life and is now being approached for advice which they are neither trained nor qualified to give. Zola has pointed out that directives issued by the medical profession have come to carry the force of moral imperatives, without their authority in this respect being challenged. Such an approach to medicine as an institution of social control has of course been more widely adopted in the field of psychiatry, and one can also point to Navarro's important work on control (1977). As the research progressed the aspect of social control became more central to our work, and has been developed elsewhere (Barrett and Roberts, 1978).

Related to an understanding of medicine as an institution of social control is an understanding of the male domination of the profession. The fact is implicit if not explicit in the socio-logical literature on medicine. The two classics in the field of medical education demonstrate this distribution clearly. Becker's *Boys in White* (1961) encapsulates the problem in its title while Merton's (1957) work on the student physician mentions the low proportion of female doctors in the USA, but fails to seek an explanation for this. In spite of the work of Margot Jeffreys (1966), and more recently Mary Ann Elston (1976), British sociologists working in this area have frequently failed to see beyond the attitudes of the group they are studying, and have failed to describe or account for the virtual exclusion of women from all high-status posts in the profession.

More recently, however, there has been increasing interest in the training of women doctors, as shown by the 1975 conference on medical manpower (not an insignificant choice of title), and equally importantly, it has been argued by Bewley and Bewley (1975) that the rate at which women doctors drop out as a result of family obligations is not significantly higher than the rate of attrition for men doctors resulting from alchoholism, emigration, removal from the medical register, and so on.

I have drawn attention above to the fact that the literature documents higher incidences of utilisation of medical services among women than men in a random survey of the population, and a higher rate of consultation among women than men. In the research, the sociological factors which might be held to account for this difference were explored. Such previous research as has been done on this subject has tended to concentrate on the 'feminine role' (Nathanson, 1975). It may well be that the social roles posited by sociologists working in this area are Procrustean beds to which the individual must adapt or be adapted. Hence the apparent distinction between the biological sex-based account of differences in morbidity between the sexes and the one based on social roles becomes in practice of little relevance. For example, Dalton (1969) maintains that the female cycle has tremendous and wide-ranging effects on the lives and work of many girls and women and documents these in terms of impaired exam results, driving errors, days off work, increased physical and mental illness and so on. Gove and Tudor (1972) on the other hand, maintain that certain characteristics of the 'housewife's role' are conducive to mental disorders (e.g. housewives have no source of gratification outside the family, have low prestige and are unskilled, have an unstructured and 'invisible' role, and suffer from unclear role expectations). These two approaches are apparently very different, but in practice, the distinction is less clear. The role theorists do not attempt to analyse *why* housework has these characteristics and in whose interests women are drafted in and out of the secondary sector of the labour market. Clearly, any formulation of role theory which fails to present roles as symptoms of the control exercised over individuals (in this case female individuals) by powerful economic and social structural forces is inadequate. Hence although it has been indicated that the concept of illness behaviour in general, and specifically as it has been applied to women, contributed to the intellectual background of the proposed research, its limitations should be stressed.

The final category of literature in the sociology of medicine relevant both to the hypotheses and methodology of the research was a category in which one would want to list all those works in which illness and the use of medical services by specific groups within society were analysed in terms of those groups' social structural background. As a paradigm of such an account, one might cite here the classic studies of Hollingshead and Redlich (1958) in which they clearly demonstrate the significance of social class as a determining variable in the incidence and treatment of mental illness.

The work done by George Brown and his associates (Brown and Harris, 1978) on the social origins of depression among women has been extremely important, but ignores a feminist perspective despite overwhelming evidence that this might be useful. Their choice of women as a sample to be studied begs some of the questions addressed by Ann Oakley in her chapter in this collection on interviewing women. Brown and Harris write (1978, p.22):

We needed as many people as possible to agree to co-operate in what we knew would be a lengthy interview. Such an interviewing programme is expensive and one way to reduce its cost was to study women only, as they probably suffer from depression more than men. It also seemed likely that women, who are more often at home during the day, would be more willing to agree to see us for several hours.

Little work has been done from a similar perspective in terms of gender and physical illness, and in conceptualising the research and research methodology it was felt that further work was needed on the social structural analysis of medicine and research in which women would be subjects rather than objects of sociological curiosity.

Given the intellectual background, what were the specific problems we faced?

One of the practical problems, that of the hierarchical nature of the research team and the normal division of labour along gender lines discussed in the introduction, was side-stepped. Both original principal investigators are women, and an early decision was made not to apply for funds for research assistance or to have tapes transcribed by a typist. The former decision was dictated partly by the qualitative nature of the research and partly by a desire to retain full control of the data. Work on the research process has indicated that many research assistants go into the work 'blind'; there is no real training apart from experience and this might lead one to ask, as Roth (1971) has done, why it is that basic scientific work is regarded as something that can be done by untrained persons. The latter decision was taken because audio typing (as any typist will bear witness) is work of the most alienating kind and as in many types of women's work, the level of skill and concentration involved is by no means compensated for by the rates of pay. In this case we reasoned that our enthusiasm for the research would render it a less appalling task for us than for an outsider. In the event, however, whilst our transcribing of the tapes solved our particular problem, it was neither fun, nor did it help us in any way to reach a realistic resolution of the intellectual and sexual division of labour in the research process in general.

The very language in which we make distinctions between qualitative and quantitative data is, as Pauline Bart (1974) writes, not gender-neutral. She has her own solution (p.1):

> we speak of hard data as being better than soft data, hard science better than soft science, hard money better than soft money. In the fifties, one was criticised for being 'soft on communism'. This is of course a male sexual metaphor, so since discovering this, I have substituted a metaphor based on female sexual experience and refer to wet and dry data.

If the number of women employed as low-status research assistants (and the number of men working as principal investigators and analysing data) is anything to go by, women are, or are seen to be, 'better' at that kind of qualitative research that involves talking to people, and 'worse' at quantitative research, i.e. counting. As Mary Ann Elston (1977) has pointed out, one reason why women may do qualitative research is that for 'good sociological reasons' they tend to see themselves as not being very good at maths.

Possibly the relatively small number of women involved in quantitative research may provide some explanation for the inadequacy of certain statistical procedures in looking at sex differences. As David Tresemer (1975) points out (p.308):

> The major misleading assumptions about gender roles are that observed differences between the sexes are reflected in biological sex differences, that differences between the sexes are more important than similarities, that the trait of masculinity-femininity is a bipolar unidimensional, continuous normally distributed variable that is highly important and consistently viewed.

Because of the association between sex and gender and the assumption which Tresemer outlines above, one cannot help but suspect that in a good deal of work in social sciences, results which do not show gender as a neat dichotomising variable are explained away. Tresemer points to the conventional wisdom that the division between the sexes is a dichotomous one (we speak of the 'opposite' sex) and the fact that conventions within social science dictate that a finding of 'no difference' is not as significant or interesting as a finding indicating differences.

A particular problem with which any sociologist is faced concerns those statistics which are unreliable because of the second-order category schemes imposed on them, such as the registrar general's classification of occupations. This classification, all-pervasive in employment, health and other statistics, is based on the way in which mens' jobs are distributed, so that even if a researcher decides to use a woman's own occupation (rather than her husband's or father's as is traditional) as a basis for social class classification, it does not really work adequately. Why then do we go on using these secondary sources? First, perhaps, because we are fallible and our resources are finite, and second because of the deadweight of sociological tradition. Oakley (1974, p.37) ultimately defended her use of the registrar general's classification in the housework study:

> There was, however, one over-riding reason for taking the conventional approach: much of the existing literature on women's domestic roles draws attention to social class differences .... Therefore, for meaningful comparisons to be possible between my own findings and those of other researchers, social class had to be assessed in the same way.

While one can only sympathise with Oakley's dilemma, one cannot help wondering what the term 'meaningful' means in a context where the assessment on one level can be seen as problematic. In conventional terms, it puts reliability and replicability above other criteria for validity, and indeed in Oakley's childbirth study (1980), this convention is questioned (p.133) and there is a social class breakdown of her sample both by male and female occupation.

Particularly in relation to health, there is reason to suppose that a woman's own occupation may well be a better indicator of her life chances than her husband's or father's occupation, but much of the work on social class and health not only uses the husband's occupation but does not even indicate that this is problematic. Brown and Harris, for instance, in addressing themselves to social class differences in susceptibility to depression, suggest that taking a woman's past or current occupation adds 'practically nothing' to the size of the association between social class and psychiatric disorder. Thus, they not only follow the normal convention of assessment through the husband's or father's occupation, but go one step further so that in some cases, a woman is not freed from classification by her husband's occupation even after he is dead (Brown and Harris, 1978, pp.155-6):

> We classified a woman by the occupation of her husband or father if she was living with either of them, and only by her own when she was not. We made one exception. For anyone who was widowed, separated or

divorced, we used the husband's usual occupation where her economic circumstances had not apparently changed a great deal.

In our own research, although information was collected on the woman's past and present occupations and on her husband's occupation, we did not feel that these data yielded useful information in terms of social class as such. In terms of social class, the problem posed is how, within institutionalised sociology, do we break out of this vicious circle, particularly from the bottom of the credibility hierarchy. The fact that the Nuffield mobility survey failed to address the problem of the mobility of women, with the exception of Llewellyn's work discussed in chapter 6, leads one to suspect that the issue is not seen as crucial within the profession as a whole.

Millman and Moss Kanter (1975) have pointed out that some methodologies and research situations may systematically prevent the elicitation of various kinds of information and that certain methodological assumptions and techniques may limit the researcher's vision and produce questionable findings. Similarly, Gouldner (1971) reminds us that 'the use of particular methods of study implies the existence of particular assumptions about man (sic) and society' (p.28).

It was mentioned above that, at the request of the Social Science Research Council, a number of men were included in our sample although the original proposal had been to look at the health of women only. There would have been considerable difficulty in interviewing a sample of middle-aged bachelors as suggested by the sociology committee. They do not form a large enough group in the average practice to provide a sample on the same basis as the women. In addition of course, given that the title 'Mr' does not distinguish between the married and the unmarried, there would have been some difficulty in discovering who the bachelors were. Those men whom the GPs were readily able to distinguish as bachelors tended to be unsuitable for the needs of the research (e.g. homeless, alcoholic, sub-normal, etc.). The two samples of men were therefore drawn on a different basis altogether and were the *husbands* of women interviewed in two of the study practices. In these cases I wrote to the women after they had been interviewed and asked whether they would mind if I also approached their husbands for an interview. I did this largely so that the women would feel reassured that I would not break any confidences they might have made.

One can only speculate on the reasons for the SSRC's suggestion that we include men in our sample, and particularly the suggestion that they be bachelors. Were these perhaps seen as a problem group in the same way as middle-aged women, while married men represent the norm? One can only hope the suggestion is indicative of a general policy on the part of the Social Science Research Council no longer to sponsor research dealing with only one sex. Perhaps in the future, we will not see studies of organisations within which the absence of women remains unquestioned or mobility studies which include only men.

Working as a feminist as well as a professional sociologist, a central concern of the research has been to attempt to integrate a feminist theory, methodology and practice and to avoid that type of academic discourse which renders research findings inaccessible to those who do not have a background in sociology. There is little point in congratulating ourselves on the fact that the validity of interpretative data can be checked by the subjects answering back, if we are to present our work in such a way that it can only be understood by a coterie of sociologists. It is clearly of particular importance when doing research with relatively powerless groups that research findings should be presented in a way which is as clear as possible to those individuals. This raises the question of whether we do research for ourselves, for our professional colleagues or for and with the subjects of our research. Ann Oakley offers a useful resolution to this problem in her studies of housework and childbirth, both of which have produced one book for the lay reader and one for the sociologist.

Feminist research, then, is concerned not only with making women visible, but with theoretical and methodological issues, with problems of sexual divisions in the research team and the research process, and with the language of research findings and the way in which these may be used when they are published.

Becker (1971, p.134) has suggested that there is a belief among sociologists that

> some problems can be approached in a 'scientific' way while other problems, no matter how interesting or important, must either be ignored for the time being, until we devise sufficiently rigorous methods, or dealt with in ways that rely on intuition and other non-communicable gifts. If no strict set of rules and procedures exists, then either don't do it or anything goes.

There is some evidence to show that this belief does most certainly exist in respect to some of the problems outlined above, but feminist sociologists, in arguing that gender should be taken into account in theory and in practice, are arguing for more and not less vigorous methods.

The issues raised above indicate in a preliminary way some of the problems involved in working as feminists and in attempting to develop an adequate methodology in doing feminist research. Some of these issues are tackled in more depth in subsequent chapters; others require further thought and development not only by feminist sociologists but by all sociologists.

Notes

1   An earlier version of this paper and some of the research on which it is based was conducted in conjunction with Michèle Barrett, but the responsibility for this version rests with me. I am grateful to Sheila Allen, Rodney Barker, Hilary Rose, Carol Smart, Margaret Stacey and particularly Mary Ann Elston for their comments on the paper. The research which it describes was financed by the Social Science Research Council and the first version of the paper was written for an SSRC workshop on qualitative methodology which took place at the University of Warwick in the summer of 1977.
2   This quotation was drawn to my attention by Pauline Bart. I am grateful to Susan Griffin for her permission to use it.
3   Margaret Stacey has suggested that during their reproductive years women may well establish a particular relationship with and reliance upon doctors because of the medicalisation of childbirth and child rearing which has occurred over the past 50 to 100 years.

4   The term 'sociosomatic' is taken to refer to physical conditions
     which are attributable to social determinants rather than to psy-
     chological states. Hence it can be argued that social class and sexual
     divisions in society can influence not only the behaviour associated
     with illness and the demand for medical attention, but also the
     underlying physical and mental complaints. As with all social struc-
     tural determinants, the process by which basic inequalities come to
     affect individuals is largely a normative and ideological one. Because
     of this observers have tended to stress the apparent psychological
     aspect, without adequately considering the social bases of individual
     states of mind.
5   The most extensive source of data on this point is the National
     Morbidity Survey conducted jointly by the Office of Population
     Censuses and Surveys and the Royal College of General Practitioners.
6   Although the attendance rates at doctors' surgeries are higher for
     women, the rates for accident and emergency departments of hos-
     pitals are higher for men.

References

Barrett, M. and Roberts, H. (1978), 'Doctors and their Patients: the
     Social Control of Women in General Practice', in Carol and Barry
     Smart (eds), *Women, Sexuality and Social Control*, Routledge &
     Kegan Paul, London.
Bart, Pauline (1974), 'Male Views of Female Sexuality, from Freud's
     Phallacies to Fisher's Inexact Test', paper presented at the second
     national meeting, special section on Psychosomatic Obstetrics and
     Gynaecology, Key Biscayne, Florida.
Becker, Howard (1961), *Boys in White: Student Culture in Medical
     Schools*, University of Chicago Press.
Becker, Howard (1971), *Sociological Work*, Allen Lane, London.
Bewley, B.R. and Bewley, T.H. (1975), 'Hospital Doctors' Career
     Structure and Misuse of Medical Womanpower', *Lancet*, 9 August,
     pp.270–2.
Brown, George H. and Harris, Tirril (1978), *Social Origins of Depres-
     sion: A Study of Psychiatric Disorder in Women*, Tavistock, London.
Brown, R.G.S. (1976), 'Social Causes of Disease' in David Tuckett, (ed.),
     An Introduction to Medical Sociology, Tavistock, London.
Clare, Anthony (1976), *Psychiatry in Dissent*, Tavistock, London.
Dalton, Katherine (1969), *The Menstrual Cycle*, Penguin, Harmonds-
     worth.
Daniels, Arlene (1975), 'Feminist Perspectives in Sociological Research',
     in Marcia Millman and Rosabeth Moss Kanter (eds), *Another Voice*,
     Anchor Books, New York.
Dreitzel, Hans Peter (ed.) (1971), *The Social Organisation of Health*,
     Macmillan, New York.

Elston, Mary Ann (1976) 'Women in the Medical Profession. Whose Problem?' in M. Stacey, M. Reid, C. Heath and R. Dingwall (eds), *Health and the Division of Labour*, Croom Helm, London.

Elston, Mary Ann (1977), 'Towards a Non-Sexist Methodology', unpublished paper presented to the BSA Women's Caucus.

Friedan, Betty (1973), *The Feminine Mystique*, W. W. Norton, New York.

Gouldner, Alvin (1971), *The Coming Crisis of Western Sociology*, Heinemann, London.

Gove, W.R. and Tudor, J. (1972), 'The Relationship between Sex Roles, Marital Status and Mental Illness', *Social Forces*, vol. 51, pp.34–44.

Griffin, Susan (1975), *Voices*, Feminist Press, New York.

Hollingshead, A.B. and Redlich, F.C. (1958), *Social Class and Mental Illness: a Community Study*, Wiley, New York.

Jeffreys, Margot, (1966), 'Marriage, Motherhood and Medicine', *Transactions of the VI World Congress of Sociology*, vol. IV, September, International Sociological Association, pp.197–211.

Katz, Alfred (1971), 'The Social Causes of Disease', in Hans Pieter Dreitzel, *The Social Organisation of Health*, Macmillan, New York.

Merton, R.K. (1957), *The Student Physician: Introductory Studies in the Sociology of Medical Education*, Harvard University Press.

Millman, Marcia and Moss Kanter, Rosabeth (eds) (1975), *Another Voice: Feminist Perspectives on Social Life and Social Science*, Anchor Books, New York.

Nathanson, C. (1975), 'Illness and the Feminine Role', *Social Science and Medicine*, vol. 9, pp.57–62.

Navarro, V. (1977), *Medicine under Capitalism*, Croom Helm, London.

Oakley, Ann (1974), *The Sociology of Housework*, Martin Robertson, London.

Oakley, Ann (1980), *Women Confined: Towards a Sociology of Childbirth*, Martin Robertson, Oxford.

Parsons, Talcott (1964), *The Social System*, Routledge & Kegan Paul, London.

Ratoff, L. (1973), 'More Social Work for General Practice?', *Journal of the Royal College of General Practitioners*, no. 23, p.736.

Roth, Julius (1971), 'Hired Hand Research', in Howard Becker, *Sociological Work*, Allen Lane, London.

Smith, Dorothy (1974), 'Women's Perspective as a Radical Critique of Sociology', *Sociological Enquiry*, vol. 44, no. 1, pp.7–13.

Tresemer, David (1975), 'Assumption made about Gender Roles', in Marcia Millman and Rosabeth Moss Kanter, *Another Voice*, Anchor Books, New York.

Wadsworth, M.E.J. *et al.* (1971), *Health and Sickness: the Choice of Treatment, Perception of Illness and Use of Services in an Urban Community*, Tavistock, London.

Zola, Irving (1972), 'Medicine as an Institution of Social Control', *Sociological Review*, no. 4.

2

Interviewing women: a contradiction in terms

Ann Oakley

In this chapter, Ann Oakley discusses methodological problems highlighted by her research on motherhood, and in particular the gap between textbook 'recipes' for interviewing and her own experience as an interviewer. Traditional criteria for interviewing, suggests Oakley, can be summarised as, first, the admonition that the interviewing situation is a one-way process in which the interviewer elicits and receives, but does not give information. Oakley illustrates the absurdity of this situation through a discussion of the questions her respondents 'asked back'. Second, textbooks advise interviewers to adopt an attitude towards interviewees which allocates the latter a narrow and objectified function as data. Third, interviews are seen as having no personal meaning in terms of social interaction, so that their meaning tends to be confined to their statistical comparability with other interviews and the data obtained from them.

Oakley suggests that each of these paradigms of traditional interviewing practice creates problems for feminist interviewers whose primary orientation is towards the validation of women's subjective experiences as women and as people, and illustrates the lack of fit between theory and practice in this area.

Interviewing is rather like marriage: everybody knows what it is, an awful lot of people do it, and yet behind each closed front door there is a world of secrets. Despite the fact that much of modern sociology could justifiably be considered 'the science of the interview' (Benney and Hughes, 1970, p.190), very few sociologists who employ interview data actually bother to describe in detail the process of interviewing itself. The conventions of research reporting require them to offer such information as how many interviews were done and how many were not done; the length of time the interviews lasted; whether the questions were asked following some standardised format or not; and how the information was recorded. Some issues on which research reports do not usually comment are: social/personal characteristics of those doing the interviewing; interviewees' feelings about being interviewed and about the interview; interviewers' feelings about interviewees; and quality of interviewer–interviewee interaction; hospitality offered by interviewees to interviewers; attempts by interviewees to use interviewers as sources of information; and the extension of interviewer–interviewee encounters into more broadly-based social relationships.

I shall argue in this chapter that social science researchers' awareness of those aspects of interviewing which are 'legitimate' and 'illegitimate' from the viewpoint of inclusion in research reports reflect their embeddedness in a particular research protocol. This protocol assumes a predominantly masculine model of sociology and society. The relative undervaluation of women's models has led to an unreal theoretical characterisation of the interview as a means of gathering sociological data which cannot and does not work in practice. This lack of fit between the theory and practice of interviewing is especially likely to come to the fore when a feminist interviewer is interviewing women (who may or may not be feminists).

Interviewing: a masculine paradigm?

Let us consider first what the methodology textbooks say about interviewing. First, and most obviously, an interview is a way of finding out about people. 'If you want an answer, ask a question . . . . The asking of questions is the main source of social scientific information about everyday behaviour' (Shipman, 1972, p.76). According to Johan Galtung (1967, p.149):

> The survey method . . . has been indispensable in gaining information about the human conditions and new insights in social theory.
>   The reasons for the success of the survey method seem to be two:
> (1) *theoretically relevant* data are obtained (2) they are amenable to *statistical treatment*, which means (a) the use of the powerful tools of correlation analysis and multi-variate analysis to test substantive relationships, and (b) the tools of statistical tests of hypotheses about generalizability from samples to universes.

Interviewing, which is one[1] means of conducting a survey is essentially a conversation, 'merely one of the many ways in which two people talk to one another' (Benney and Hughes, 1970, p.191), but it is also, significantly, an *instrument* of data collection: 'the interviewer is really a tool or an instrument'[2] (Goode and Hatt, 1952, p.185). As Benny and Hughes express it, (1970, pp.196–7):

> Regarded as an information-gathering tool, the interview is designed to minimise the local, concrete, immediate circumstances of the particular encounter – including the respective personalities of the participants – and to emphasise only those aspects that can be kept general enough and demonstrable enough to be counted. As an encounter between these two particular people the typical interview has no meaning; it is conceived in a framework of other, comparable meetings between other couples, each recorded in such fashion that elements of communication in common can be easily isolated from more idiosyncratic qualities.

Thus an interview is 'not simply a conversation. It is, rather, a pseudo-conversation. In order to be successful, it must have all the warmth and personality exchange of a conversation with the clarity and guidelines of scientific searching' (Goode and Hatt, 1952, p.191). This requirement means that the interview must be seen as 'a specialised pattern of verbal interaction — initiated for a specific purpose, and focussed on some specific content areas, with consequent elimination of extraneous material' (Kahn and Cannell, 1957, p.16).

The motif of successful interviewing is 'be friendly but not too friendly'. For the contradiction at the heart of the text-book paradigm is that interviewing necessitates the manipulation of interviewees as objects of study/sources of data, but this can only be achieved via a certain amount of humane treatment. If the interviewee doesn't believe he/she is being kindly and sympathetically treated by the interviewer, then he/she will not consent to be studied and will not come up with the desired information. A balance must then be struck between the warmth required to generate 'rapport' and the detachment necessary to see the interviewee as an object under surveillance; walking this tightrope means, not surprisingly, that 'interviewing is not easy' (Denzin, 1970, p.186), although mostly the textbooks do support the idea that it *is* possible to be a perfect interviewer and both to get reliable and valid data and make interviewees believe they are not simple statistics-to-be. It is just a matter of following the rules.

A major preoccupation in the spelling out of the rules is to counsel potential interviewers about where necessary friendliness ends and unwarranted involvement begins. Goode and Hatt's statement on this topic quoted earlier, for example, continues (1952, p.191):

Consequently, the interviewer cannot merely lose him-self[3] in being friendly. He must introduce himself as though beginning a conversation but from the beginning the additional element of respect, of professional competence, should be maintained. Even the beginning student will make this attempt, else he will find himself merely 'maintaining rapport', while failing to penetrate the clichés of contradictions of the respondent. Further he will find that his own confidence is lessened, if his only goal is to maintain friendliness. He is a professional researcher in this situation and he must demand and obtain respect for the task he is trying to perform.

Claire Selltiz and her colleagues give a more explicit recipe. They say (1965, p.576):

The interviewer's manner should be friendly, courteous, conversational and unbiased. He should be neither too grim nor too effusive; neither too talkative nor too timid. The idea should be to put the respondent at ease, so that he[4] will talk freely and fully . . . . [Hence,] A brief remark about the weather, the family pets, flowers or children will often serve to break the ice. Above all, an informal, conversational interview is dependent upon a thorough mastery by the interviewer of the actual questions in his schedule. He should be familiar enough with them to ask them conversationally, rather than read them stiffly; and he should know what questions are coming next, so there will be no awkward pauses while he studies the questionnaire.

C.A. Moser, in an earlier text, (1958, pp.187–8, 195) advises of the dangers of 'overrapport'.

Some interviewers are no doubt better than others at establishing what the psychologists call 'rapport' and some may even be too good at it — the National Opinion Research Centre Studies[5] found slightly less satisfactory results from the . . . sociable interviewers who are 'fascinated by people' . . . there is something to be said for the interviewer who, while friendly and interested does not get too emotionally involved with the respondent and his problems. Interviewing on most surveys is a fairly straightforward job, not one calling for exceptional industry, charm or tact. What one asks is that the interviewer's personality should be neither over-aggressive nor over-sociable. Pleasantness and a business-like nature is the ideal combination.

'Rapport', a commonly used but ill-defined term, does not mean in this context what the dictionary says it does ('a sympathetic relationship', *O.E.D.*) but the acceptance by the interviewee of the interviewer's research goals and the interviewee's active search to help the interviewer in providing the relevant information. The person who is interviewed has a passive role in adapting to the definition of the situation offered by the person doing the interviewing. The person doing the interviewing must actively and continually construct the 'respondent' (a telling name) as passive. Another way to phrase this is to say that both interviewer and interviewee must be 'socialised' into the correct interviewing behaviour (Sjoberg and Nett, 1968, p.210):

> it is essential not only to train scientists to construct carefully worded questions and draw respresentative samples but also to educate the public to respond to questions on matters of interest to scientists and to do so in a manner advantageous for scientific analysis. To the extent that such is achieved, a common bond is established between interviewer and interviewee. [However,] It is not enough for the scientist to understand the world of meaning of his informants; if he is to secure valid data via the structured interview, respondents must be socialised into answering questions in proper fashion.

One piece of behaviour that properly socialised respondents do not engage in is asking questions back. Although the textbooks do not present any evidence about the extent to which interviewers do find in practice that this happens, they warn of its dangers and in the process suggest some possible strategies of avoidance: 'Never provide the interviewee with any formal indication of the interviewer's beliefs and values. If the informant[6] poses a question . . . parry it' (Sjoberg and Nett, 1968, p.212). 'When asked what you mean and think, tell them you are here to learn, not to pass any judgement, that the situation is very complex' (Galtung 1967, p.161). 'If he (the interviewer) should be asked for his views, he should laugh off the request with the remark that his job at the moment is to get opinions, not to have them' (Selltiz *et al.*, 1965, p.576), and so on. Goode and Hatt (1952, p.198) offer the most detailed advice on this issue:

> What is the interviewer to do, however, if the respondent really wants information? Suppose the interviewee does answer the question but than asks for the opinions of the interviewer. Should he give his honest opinion, or an opinion which he thinks the interviewee wants? In most cases, the rule remains that he is there to obtain information and to focus on the respondent, not himself. Usually, a few simple phrases will shift the emphasis back to the respondent. Some which have been fairly successful are 'I guess I haven't thought enough about it to give a good answer right now', 'Well, right now, your opinions are more important than mine', and 'If you really want to know what I think, I'll be honest and tell you in a moment, after we've finished the interview.' Sometimes the diversion can be accomplished by a head-shaking gesture which suggests 'That's a hard one!' while continuing with the interview. In short, the interviewer must avoid the temptation to express his own views, even if given the opportunity.

Of course the reason why the interviewer must pretend not to have opinions (or to be possessed of information the interviewee wants) is because behaving otherwise might 'bias' the interview. 'Bias' occurs when there are systematic differences between interviewers in the way interviews are conducted, with resulting differences in the data produced. Such bias clearly invalidates the scientific claims of the research, since the question of which information might be coloured by interviewees' responses to interviewers' attitudinal stances and which is independent of this 'contamination' cannot be settled in any decisive way.

The paradigm of the social research interview prompted in the methodology textbooks does, then, emphasise (a) its status as a mechanical instrument of data-collection; (b) its function as a specialised form of conversation in which one person asks the questions and another gives the answers; (c) its characterisation of interviewees as essentially passive individuals, and (d) its reduction of interviewers to a question asking and rapport-promoting role. Actually, two separate typifications of the interviewer are prominent in the literature, though the disjunction between the two is never commented on. In one the interviewer is 'a combined phonograph and recording system' (Rose, 1945, p.143); the job of the interviewer 'is fundamentally that of a reporter, not an evangelist, a curiosity-seeker, or a debater' (Selltiz *et al.*, 1965, p.576). It is important to note that while the interviewer must treat the interviewee as an object or data-producing machine which, when handled correctly will function properly, the interviewer herself/himself has the same status from the point of view of the person/people, institution or corporation conducting the research. Both interviewer and interviewee are thus depersonalised participants in the research process.

The second typification of interviewers in the methodology literature is that of the interviewer as psychoanalyst. The interviewer's relationship to the interviewee is hierarchical and it is the body of expertise possessed by the interviewer that allows the interview to be successfully conducted. Most crucial in this exercise is the interviewer's use of non-directive comments and probes to encourage a free association of ideas which reveals whatever truth the research has been set up to uncover. Indeed, the term 'nondirective interview' is derived directly from the language of psychotherapy and carries the logic of interviewer-impersonality to its extreme (Selltiz *et al.*, 1965, p.268):

> Perhaps the most typical remarks made by the interviewer in a nondirective interview are: 'You feel that . . .' or 'Tell me more' or 'Why?' or 'Isn't that interesting?' or simply 'Uh huh'. The nondirective interviewer's function is primarily to serve as a catalyst to a comprehensive expression of the subject's feelings and beliefs and of the frame of reference within which his feelings and beliefs take on personal significance. To achieve this result, the interviewer must create a completely permissive atmosphere, in which the subject is free to express himself without fear of disapproval, admonition or dispute and without advice from the interviewer.

Sjoberg and Nett spell out the premises of the free association method (1968, p.211):

> the actor's (interviewee's) mental condition (is) . . .
> confused and difficult to grasp. Frequently the actor
> himself does not know what he believes; he may be so
> 'immature' that he cannot perceive or cope with his own
> subconscious thought patterns . . . the interviewer must
> be prepared to follow the interviewee through a jungle
> of meandering thought ways if he is to arrive at the per-
> son's true self.

It seems clear that both psychoanalytic and mechanical typifications of the interviewer and, indeed, the entire paradigmatic representation of 'proper' interviews in the methodology textbooks, owe a great deal more to a masculine social and sociological vantage point than to a feminine one. For example, the paradigm of the 'proper' interview appeals to such values as objectivity, detachment, hierarchy and 'science' as an important cultural activity which takes priority over people's more individualised concerns. Thus the errors of poor interviewing comprise subjectivity, involvement, the 'fiction'[7] of equality and an undue concern with the ways in which people are not statistically comparable. This polarity of 'proper' and 'improper' interviewing is an almost classical representation of the widespread gender stereotyping which has been shown, in countless studies, to occur in modern industrial civilisations (see for example Bernard, 1975, part I; Fransella and Frost, 1977; Griffiths and Saraga, 1979; Oakley, 1972; Sayers, 1979). Women are characterised as sensitive, intuitive, incapable of objectivity and emotional detachment and as immersed in the business of making and sustaining personal relationships. Men are though superior through their capacity for rationality and scientific objectivity and are thus seen to be possessed of an instrumental orientation in their relationships with others. Women are the exploited, the abused; they are unable to exploit others through the 'natural' weakness of altruism — a quality which is also their strength as wives, mothers and housewives. Conversely, men find it easy to exploit, although it is most important that any exploitation be justified in the name of some broad political or economic ideology ('the end justifies the means').

Feminine and masculine psychology in patriarchal societies is the psychology of subordinate and dominant social groups. The tie between women's irrationality and heightened sensibility on the one hand and their materially disadvantaged position on the other is, for example, also to be found in the case of ethnic minorities. The psychological characteristics of subordinates 'form a certain familiar cluster: submissiveness, passivity, docility, dependency, lack of initiative, inability to act, to decide, to think and the like. In general, this cluster includes qualities more characteristic of children than adults — immaturity, weakness and helplessness. If subordinates adopt these characteristics, they are considered well adjusted' (Miller, 1976, p.7). It is no accident that the methodology textbooks (with one notable exception) (Moser, 1958)[8] refer to the interviewer as male. Although not all interviewees are referred to as female, there are a number of references to 'housewives' as the kind of people interviewers are most likely to meet in the course of their work (for example Goode and Hatt, 1952, p.189). Some of what Jean Baker Miller has to say about the relationship between dominant and subordinate groups would appear to be relevant to this paradigmatic interviewer–interviewee relationship (Miller, 1976, pp.6–8):

> A dominant group, inevitably, has the greatest influence in determining a culture's overall outlook — its philosophy, morality, social theory and even its science. The dominant group, thus, legitimizes the unequal relationship and incorporates it into society's guiding concepts. . . .
>
> Inevitably the dominant group is the model for 'normal human relationships'. It then becomes 'normal' to treat others destructively and to derogate them, to obscure the truth of what you are doing by creating false explanations and to oppose actions toward equality. In short, if one's identification is with the dominant group, it is 'normal' to continue in this pattern. . . .
>
> It follows from this that dominant groups generally

do not like to be told about or even quietly reminded of the existence of inequality. 'Normally' they can avoid awareness because their explanation of the relationship becomes so well integrated *in other terms*; they can even believe that both they and the subordinate group share the same interests and, to some extent, a common experience.. . .

Clearly, inequality has created a state of conflict. Yet dominant groups will tend to suppress conflict. They will see any questioning of the 'normal' situation as threatening; activities by subordinates in this direction will be perceived with alarm. Dominants are usually convinced that the way things are is right and good, not only for them but especially for the subordinates. All morality confirms this view and all social structure sustains it.

To paraphrase the relevance of this to the interviewer–interviewee relationship we could say that: interviewers define the role of interviewees as subordinates; extracting information is more to be valued than yielding it; the convention of interviewer-interviewee hierarchy is a rationalisation of inequality; what is good for interviewers is not necessarily good for interviewees.

Another way to approach this question of the masculinity of the 'proper' interview is to observe that a sociology of feelings and emotion does not exist. Sociology mirrors society in not looking at social interaction from the viewpoint of women (Smith, 1979; Oakley, 1974, chapter 1). While eveyone has feelings, 'Our society defines being cognitive, intellectual or rational dimensions of experience as superior to being emotional or sentimental. (Significantly, the terms "emotional" and "sentimental" have come to connote excessive or degenerate forms of feeling). Through the prism of our technological and rationalistic culture, we are led to perceive and feel emotions as some irrelevancy or impediment to getting things done.' Hence their role in interviewing. But 'Another reason for sociologists' neglect of emotions may be the discipline's attempt to be recognised as a "real science" and the consequent need to focus on the most objective and measurable features of social life. This coincides with the values of the traditional "male culture"' (Hochschild, 1975, p.281).

Getting involved with the people you inteview is doubly bad: it jeopardises the hard-won status of sociology as a science and is indicative of a form of personal degeneracy.

Women interviewing women: or objectifying your sister

Before I became an interviewer I had read what the textbooks said interviewing ought to be. However, I found it very difficult to realise the prescription in practice, in a number of ways which I describe below. It was these practical difficulties which led me to take a new look at the textbook paradigm. In the rest of this chapter the case I want to make is that when a feminist interviews women: (1) use of prescribed interviewing practice is morally indefensible; (2) general and irreconcilable contradictions at the heart of the textbook paradigm are exposed; and (3) it becomes clear that, in most cases, the goal of finding out about people through interviewing is best achieved when the relationship of interviewer and interviewee is non-hierarchical and when the interviewer is prepared to invest his or her own personal identity in the relationship.

Before arguing the general case I will briefly mention some relevant aspects of my own interviewing experience. I have interviewed several hundred women over a period of some ten years, but it was the most recent research project, one concerned with the transition to motherhood, that particularly highlighted problems in the conventional interviewing recipe. Salient features of this research were that it involved repeated interviewing of a sample of women during a critical phase in their lives (in fact 55 women were interviewed four times; twice in pregnancy and twice afterwards and the average total period of interviewing was 9.4 hours.) It included for some[9] my attendance at the most critical point in this phase: the birth of the baby. The research was preceded by nine months of participant observation chiefly in the hospital setting of interactions between mothers or mothers-to-be and medical people. Although I had a research assistant to help me, I myself did the bulk of the interviewing — 178 interviews over a period of some 12 months.[10] The project was my idea[11] and the analysis and writing up of the data was entirely my responsibility.

My difficulties in interviewing women were of two main kinds. First, they asked me a great many questions. Second, repeated interviewing over this kind of period and involving the intensely personal experiences of pregnancy, birth and motherhood, established a rationale of personal involvement I found it problematic and ultimately unhelpful to avoid.

Asking questions back

Analysing[12] the tape-recorded interviews I had conducted, I listed 878 questions that interviewees had asked me at some point in the interviewing process. Three-quarters of these (see Table 2.1) were requests for information (e.g. 'Who will

Table 2.1 *Questions interviewees asked (total 878), Transition to Motherhood Project (percentages)*

Information requests	76
Personal questions	15
Questions about the research	6
Advice questions	4

deliver my baby?' 'How do you cook an egg for a baby?') Fifteen per cent were questions about me, my experiences or attitudes in the area of reproduction ('Have you got any children?' 'Did you breast feed?'); 6 per cent were questions about the research ('Are you going to write a book?'. 'Who pays you for doing this?'), and 4 per cent were more directly requests for advice on a particular matter ('How long should you wait for sex after childbirth?' 'Do you think my baby's got too many clothes on?'). Table 2.2 goes into more detail about the topics on which interviewees wanted information. The largest category of questions concerned medical procedures: for example, how induction of labour is done, and whether all women attending a particular hospital[13] are given episiotomies. The second-largest category related to infant care or development: for example, 'How do you clean a

Table 2.2 *Interviewees' requests for information (total 664), Transition to Motherhood Project (percentages)*

Medical procedures	31
Organisational procedures	19
Physiology of reproduction	15
Baby care/development/feeding	21
Other	15

baby's nails?' 'When do babies sleep through the night?' Third, there were questions about organisational procedures in the institutional settings where antenatal or delivery care was done; typical questions were concerned with who exactly would be doing antenatal care and what the rules are for husbands' attendance at delivery. Last, there were questions about the physiology of reproduction; for example 'Why do some women need caesareans?' and (from one very frightened mother-to-be) 'Is it right that the baby doesn't come out of the same hole you pass water out of?'

It would be the understatement of all time to say that I found it very difficult to avoid answering these questions as honestly and fully as I could. I was faced, typically, with a woman who was quite anxious about the fate of herself and her baby, who found it either impossible or extremely difficult to ask questions and receive satisfactory answers from the medical staff with whom she came into contact, and who saw me as someone who could not only reassure but inform.[14] I felt that I was asking a great deal from these women in the way of time, co-operation and hospitality at a stage in their lives when they had every reason to exclude strangers altogether in order to concentrate on the momentous character of the experiences being lived through. Indeed, I *was* asking a great deal — not only 9.4 hours of interviewing time but confidences on highly personal matters such as sex and money and 'real' (i.e. possibly negative or ambivalent) feelings about babies, husbands, etc. I was, in addition, asking some of the women to allow me to witness them in the highly personal act of giving birth. Although the pregnancy interviews did not have to compete with the demands of motherhood for time,

90 per cent of the women were employed when first interviewed and 76 per cent of the first interviews had to take
place in the evenings. Although I had timed the first postnatal
interview (at about five weeks postpartum) to occur after the
disturbances of very early motherhood, for many women it
was nevertheless a stressful and busy time. And all this in the
interests of 'science' or for some book that might possibly
materialise out of the research — a book which many of the
women interviewed would not read and none would profit
from directly (though they hoped that they would not lose
too much).

The transition to friendship?

In a paper on 'Collaborative Interviewing and Interactive
Research', Laslett and Rapoport (1975) discuss the advantages
and disadvantages of repeated interviewing. They say (p.968)
that the gain in terms of collecting more information in greater
depth than would otherwise be possible is partly made by
'being responsive to, rather than seeking to avoid, respondent
reactions to the interview situation and experience'. This sort
of research is deemed by them 'interactive'. The principle of
a hierarchical relationship between interviewer and interviewee
is not adhered to and 'an attempt is made to generate a collaborative approach to the research which engages both the interviewer and respondent in a joint enterprise'. Such an
approach explicitly does not seek to minimise the personal
involvement of the interviewer but as Rapoport and Rapoport
(1976, p.31) put it, relies 'very much on the formulation of a
relationship between interviewer and interviewee as an important element in achieving the quality of the information . . .
required'.[15]

As Laslett and Rapoport note, repeated interviewing is not
much discussed in the methodological literature: the paradigm
is of an interview as a 'one-off' affair. Common sense would
suggest that an ethic of detachment on the interviewer's part
is much easier to maintain where there is only one meeting
with the interviewee (and the idea of a 'one-off' affair rather
than a long-term relationship is undoubtedly closer to the
traditional masculine world view I discussed earlier).

In terms of my experience in the childbirth project, I found that interviewees very often took the initiative in defining the interviewer–interviewee relationship as something which existed beyond the limits of question-asking and answering. For example, they did not only offer the minimum hospitality of accommodating me in their homes for the duration of the interview: at 92 per cent of the interviews I was offered tea, coffee or some other drink; 14 per cent of the women also offered me a meal on at least one occasion. As Table 2.1 suggests, there was also a certain amount of interest in my own situation. What sort of person was I and how did I come to be interested in this subject?

In some cases these kind of 'respondent' reactions were evident at the first interview. More often they were generated after the second interview and an important factor here was probably the timing of the interviews. There was an average of 20 weeks between interviews 1 and 2, an average of 11 weeks between interviews 2 and 3 and an average of 15 weeks between interviews 3 and 4. Between the first two interviews most of the women were very busy. Most were still employed and had the extra work of preparing equipment/clothes/a room for the baby — which sometimes meant moving house. Between interviews 2 and 3 most were not out at work and, sensitised by the questions I had asked in the first two interviews to my interest in their birth experiences, probably began to associate me in a more direct way with their experiences of the transition to motherhood. At interview 2 I gave them all a stamped addressed postcard on which I asked them to write the date of their baby's birth so I would know when to re-contact them for the first postnatal interview. I noticed that this was usually placed in a prominent position (for example on the mantlepiece), to remind the woman or her husband to complete it and it probably served in this way as a reminder of my intrusion into their lives. One illustration of this awareness comes from the third interview with Mary Rosen, a 25-year-old exhibition organiser: 'I thought of you after he was born, I thought she'll *never* believe it — a six-hour labour, a 9lb 6 oz baby and *no* forceps — and all without an epidural, although I had said to you that I wanted one.' Sixty two per cent of the women expressed a sustained and quite detailed interest in the research; they wanted to know its goals, any proposed methods for disseminating its findings, how I had come to think of it in the first place, what the attitudes of doctors I had met or collaborated with were to it and so forth. Some of the women took the initiative in contacting me to arrange the second or a subsequent interview, although I had made it clear that I would get in touch with them. Several rang up to report particularly important pieces of information about their antenatal care — in one case a distressing encounter with a doctor who told a woman keen on natural childbirth that this was 'for animals: in this hospital we give epidurals'; in another case to tell me of an ultrasound result that changed the expected date of delivery. Several also got in touch to correct or add to things they had said during an interview — for instance, one contacted me several weeks after the fourth interview to explain that she had had an emergency appendicectomy five days after my visit and that her physical symptoms at the time could have affected some of her responses to the questions I asked.

Arguably, these signs of interviewees' involvement indicated their acceptance of the goals of the research project rather than any desire to feel themselves participating in a personal relationship with me. Yet the research was presented to them as *my* research in which I had a personal interest, so it is not likely that a hard and fast dividing line between the two was drawn. One index of their and my reactions to our joint participation in the repeated interviewing situation is that some four years after the final interview I am still in touch with more than a third of the women I interviewed. Four have become close friends, several others I visit occasionally, and the rest write or telephone when they have something salient to report such as the birth of another child.

A feminist interviews women

Such responses as I have described on the part of the interviewees to participation in research, particularly that involving repeated interviewing, are not unknown, although they are almost certainly under-reported. It could be suggested that the reasons why they were so pronounced in the research project discussed here is because of the attitudes of the interviewer — i.e. the women were reacting to my own evident wish for a relatively intimate and non-hierarchical relationship. While I was careful not to take direct initiatives in this direction, I certainly set out to convey to the people whose cooperation I was seeking the fact that I did not intend to exploit either them or the information they gave me. For instance, if the interview clashed with the demands of housework and motherhood I offered to, and often did, help with the work that had to be done. When asking the women's permission to record the interview, I said that no one but me would ever listen to the tapes; in mentioning the possibility of publications arising out of the research I told tham that their names and personal details would be changed and I would, if they wished, send them details of any such publications, and so forth. The attitude I conveyed could have had some influence in encouraging the women to regard me as a friend rather than purely as a data-gatherer.

The pilot interviews, together with my previous experience of interviewing women, led me to decide that when I was asked questions I would answer them. The practice I followed was to answer all personal questions and questions about the research as fully as was required. For example, when two women asked if I had read their hospital case notes I said I had, and when one of them went on to ask what reason was given in these notes for her forceps delivery, I told her what the notes said. On the emotive issue of whether I experienced childbirth as painful (a common topic of conversation) I told them that I did find it so but that in my view it was worth it to get a baby at the end. Advice questions I also answered fully but made it clear when I was using my own experiences of motherhood as the basis for advice. I also referred women requesting advice to the antenatal and childbearing advice literature or to health visitors, GPs, etc. when appropriate — though the women usually made it clear that it was my opinion in particular they were soliciting. When asked for information I gave it if I could or, again, referred the questioner to an appropriate medical or non-medical authority. Again, the way I responded to interviewee's questions probably encouraged them to regard me as more than an instrument of data-collection.

Dissecting my practice of interviewing further, there were three principal reasons why I decided not to follow the text-book code of ethics with regard to interviewing women. First, I did not regard it as reasonable to adopt a purely exploitative attitude to interviewees as sources of data. My involvement in the women's movement in the early 1970s and the rebirth of feminism in an academic context had led me, along with many others, to re-assess society and sociology as masculine paradigms and to want to bring about change in the traditional cultural and academic treatment of women. 'Sisterhood', a somewhat nebulous and problematic, but nevertheless important, concept,[16] certainly demanded that women re-evaluate the basis of their relationships with one another.

The dilemma of a feminist interviewer interviewing women could be summarised by considering the practical application of some of the strategies recommended in the textbooks for meeting interviewee's questions. For example, these advise that such questions as 'Which hole does the baby come out of?' 'Does an epidural ever paralyse women?' and 'Why is it dangerous to leave a small baby alone in the house?' should be met with such responses from the interviewer as 'I guess I haven't thought enough about it to give a good answer right now,' or 'a head-shaking gesture which suggests "that's a hard one" ' (Goode and Hatt, quoted above). Also recommended is laughing off the request with the remark that 'my job at the moment is to get opinions, not to have them' (Selltiz *et al.*, quoted above).

A second reason for departing from conventional inter-viewing ethics was that I regarded sociological research as an essential way of giving the subjective situation of women greater visibility not only in sociology, but, more importantly, in society, than it has traditionally had. Interviewing women was, then, a strategy for documenting women's own accounts of their lives. What *was* important was not taken-for-granted sociological assumptions about the role of the interviewer but a new awareness of the interviewer as an instrument for pro-moting a sociology for women[17] — that is, as a tool for making possible the articulated and recorded commentary of women on the very personal business of being female in a patriarchal capitalist society. Note that the formulation of the interviewer role has changed dramatically from being a data-collecting instrument for researchers to being a data-collecting instrument for those whose lives are being researched. Such a reformulation is enhanced where the interviewer is also the researcher. It is not coincidental that in the methodological literature the paradigm of the research process is essentially disjunctive, i.e. researcher and interviewer functions are typically performed by different individuals.

A third reason why I undertook the childbirth research with a degree of scepticism about how far traditional percepts of interviewing could, or should, be applied in practice was because I had found, in my previous interviewing experiences, that an attitude of refusing to answer questions or offer any kind of personal feedback was not helpful in terms of the traditional goal of promoting 'rapport'. A different role, that could be termed 'no intimacy without reciprocity', seemed especially important in longitudinal in-depth interviewing. Without feeling that the interviewing process offered some personal satisfaction to them, interviewees would not be prepared to continue after the first interview. This involves being sensitive not only to those questions that are asked (by either party) but to those that are not asked. The interviewee's definition of the interview is important.

The success of this method cannot, of course, be judged from the evidence I have given so far. On the question of the rapport established in the Transition to Motherhood research I offer the following cameo:

A.O.: 'Did you have any questions you wanted to ask but didn't when you last went to the hospital?'

M.C.: 'Er, I don't know how to put this really. After sexual intercourse I had some bleeding, three times, only a few drops and I didn't tell the hospital because I didn't know how to put it to them. It worried me first off, as soon as I saw it I cried. I don't know if I'd be able to tell them. You see, I've also got a sore down there and a discharge and you know I wash there lots of times

a day. You think I should tell the hospital; I
could never speak to my own doctor about it.
You see I feel like this but I can talk to you
about it and I can talk to my sister about it.'

More generally the quality and depth of the information given
to me by the women I interviewed can be assessed in *Becoming
a Mother* (Oakley, 1979), the book arising out of the research
which is based almost exclusively on interviewee accounts.

So far as interviewees' reactions to being interviewed are
concerned, I asked them at the end of the last interview the
question, 'Do you feel that being involved in this research —
my coming to see you — has affected your experience of becoming a mother in any way?' Table 2.3 shows the answers.

Table 2.3 *'Has the research affected your experience of
becoming a mother?' (percentages)*

No	27
Yes:	73
Thought about it more	30
Found it reassuring	25
A relief to talk	25
Changed attitudes/behaviour	7

*Percentages do not add up to 100% because some women gave more than one
answer.

Nearly three-quarters of the women said that being interviewed
had affected them and the three most common forms this influence took were in leading them to reflect on their experiences more than they would otherwise have done; in reducing
the level of their anxiety and/or in reassuring them of their
normality; and in giving a valuable outlet for the verbalisation
of feelings. None of those who thought being interviewed
had affected them regarded this affect as negative. There were
many references to the 'therapeutic' effect of talking: 'getting
it out of your system'. (It was generally felt that husbands,
mothers, friends, etc., did not provide a sufficiently sympathetic or interested audience for a detailed recounting of

the experiences and difficulties of becoming a mother.) It is perhaps important to note here that one of the main conclusions of the research was that there is a considerable discrepancy between the expectations and the reality of the different aspects of motherhood — pregnancy, childbirth, the emotional relationship of mother and child, the work of childrearing. A dominant metaphor used by interviewees to describe their reactions to this hiatus was 'shock'. In this sense, a process of emotional recovery is endemic in the normal transition to motherhood and there is a general need for some kind of 'therapeutic listener' that is not met within the usual circle of family and friends.

On the issue of co-operation, only 2 out of 82 women contacted initially about the research actually refused to take part in it,[18] making a refusal rate of 2 per cent which is extremely low. Once the interviewing was under way only one woman voluntarily dropped out (because of marital problems); an attrition from 66 at interview 1 to 55 at interview 4 was otherwise accounted for by miscarriage, moves, etc. All the women who were asked if they would mind me attending the birth said they didn't mind and all got in touch either directly or indirectly through their husbands when they started labour. The postcards left after interview 2 for interviewees to return after the birth were all completed and returned.

Is a 'proper' interview ever possible?

Hidden amongst the admonitions on how to be a perfect interviewer in the social research methods manuals is the covert recognition that the goal of perfection is actually unattainable: the contradiction between the need for 'rapport' and the requirement of between-interview comparability cannot be solved. For example, Dexter (1956, p.156) following Paul (1954), observes that the pretence of neutrality on the interviewer's part is counterproductive: participation demands alignment. Selltiz *et al.* (1965, p.583) says that

Much of what we call interviewer bias can more correctly be described as interviewer *differences*, which are

inherent in the fact that interviewers are human beings
and not machines and that they do not work identically.

Richardson and his colleagues in their popular textbook on
interviewing (1965, p.129) note that

> Although gaining and maintaining satisfactory participa-
> tion is never the primary objective of the interviewer, it is
> so intimately related to the quality and quantity of the in-
> formation sought that the interviewer must always main-
> tain a dual concern: for the quality of his respondent's
> participation and for the quality of the information being
> sought. Often ... these qualities are independent of each
> other and occasionally they may be mutually exclusive.

It is not hard to find echoes of this point of view in the
few accounts of the actual process of interviewing that do
exist. For example, Zweig, in his study of *Labour, Life and
Poverty*, (1949, pp.1–2)

> dropped the idea of a questionnaire or formal verbal
> questions ... instead I had casual talks with working-
> class men on an absolutely equal footing ...
>   I made many friends and some of them paid me a
> visit afterwards or expressed a wish to keep in touch with
> me. Some of them confided their troubles to me and I
> often heard the remark: 'Strangely enough, I have never
> talked about that to anybody else'. They regarded my
> interest in their way of life as a sign of sympathy and
> understanding rarely shown to them even in the inner
> circle of their family. I never posed as somebody superior
> to them, or as a judge of their actions but as one of
> them.

Zweig defended his method on the grounds that telling people they were objects of study met with 'an icy reception' and
that finding out about other peoples' lives is much more readily
done on a basis of friendship than in a formal interview.
    More typically and recently, Marie Corbin, the interviewer
for the Pahls' study of *Managers and their Wives*, commented

in an Appendix to the book of that name (Corbin, 1971, pp.303–5):

> Obviously the exact type of relationship that is formed between an interviewer and the people being interviewed is something that the interviewer cannot control entirely, even though the nature of this relationship and how the interviewees classify the interviewer will affect the kinds of information given . . . simply because I am a woman and a wife I shared interests with the other wives and this helped to make the relationship a relaxed one.

Corbin goes on:

> In these particular interviews I was conscious of the need to establish some kind of confidence with the couples if the sorts of information required were to be forth-coming . . . . In theory it should be possible to establish confidence simply by courtesy towards and interest in the interviewees. In practice it can be difficult to spend eight hours in a person's home, share their meals and listen to their problems and at the same time remain polite, detached and largely uncommunicative. I found the balance between prejudicing the answers to questions which covered almost every aspect of the couples' lives, establishing a relationship that would allow the inter-views to be successful and holding a civilised conversation over dinner to be a very precarious one.

Discussing research on copper mining on Bougainville Island, Papua New Guinea, Alexander Mamak describes his growing consciousness of the political context in which research is done (1978, p.176):

> as I became increasingly aware of the unequal relation-ship existing between management and the union, I found myself becoming more and more emotionally involved in the proceedings. I do not believe this reaction is unusual since, in the words of the wellknown black sociologist Nathan Hare, 'If one is truly cognizant of

adverse circumstances, he would be expected, through the process of reason, to experience some emotional response'.

And, a third illustration of this point, Dorothy Hobson's account of her research on housewives' experiences of social isolation contains the following remarks (1978, pp.80–1):

> The method of interviewing in a one-to-one situation requires some comment. What I find most difficult is to resist commenting in a way which may direct the answers which the women give to my questions. However, when the taped interview ends we usually talk and then the women ask me questions about my life and family. These questions often reflect areas where they have experienced ambivalent feelings in their own replies. For example, one woman who said during the interview that she did not like being married, asked me how long I had been married and if I liked it. When I told her how long I had been married she said, 'Well I suppose you get used to it in time, I suppose I will'. In fact the informal talk after the interview often continues what the women have said during the interview.
> It is impossible to tell exactly how the women perceive me but I do not think they see me as too far removed from themselves. This may partly be because I have to arrange the interviews when my own son is at school and leave in time to collect him.[19]

As Bell and Newby (1977, pp.9–10) note 'accounts of doing sociological research are at least as valuable, both to students of sociology and its practitioners, as the exhortations to be found in the much more common textbooks on methodology'. All research is political, 'from the micropolitics of interpersonal relationships, through the politics of research units, institutions and universities, to those of government departments and finally to the state' — which is one reason why social research is not 'like it is presented and prescribed in those texts. It is infinitely more complex, messy, various and much more interesting' (Bell and Encel, 1978, p.4). The 'cookbooks' of research methods largely ignore the political context of research, although some make asides about its 'ethical dilemmas': 'Since we are all human we are all involved in what we are studying when we try to study any aspect of social relations' (Stacey, 1969, p.2); 'frequently researchers, in the course of their interviewing, establish rapport not as scientists but as human beings; yet they proceed to use this humanistically gained knowledge for scientific ends, usually without the informants' knowledge' (Sjoberg and Nett, 1968, pp.215–16).

These ethical dilemmas are generic to all research involving interviewing for reasons I have already discussed. But they are greatest where there is least social distance between the interviewer and interviewee. Where both share the same gender socialisation and critical life-experiences, social distance can be minimal. Where both interviewer and interviewee share membership of the same minority group, the basis for equality may impress itself even more urgently on the interviewer's consciousness. Mamak's comments apply equally to a feminist interviewing women (1978, p.168):

I found that my academic training in the methodological views of Western social science and its emphasis on 'scientific objectivity' conflicted with the experiences of my colonial past. The traditional way in which social science research is conducted proved inadequate for an understanding of the reality, needs and desires of the people I was researching.

Some of the reasons why a 'proper' interview is a masculine fiction are illustrated by observations from another field in which individuals try to find out about other individuals — anthropology. Evans-Pritchard reported this conversation during his early research with the Nuers of East Africa (1940, pp.12–13):

I: 'Who are you?'
Cuol: 'A man.'
I: 'What is your name?'
Cuol: 'Do you want to know my *name*?'

I: 'Yes.'

Cuol: 'You want to know *my* name?'

I: 'Yes, you have come to visit me in my tent and I would like to know who you are.'

Cuol: 'All right, I am Cuol. What is your name?'

I: 'My name is Pritchard.'

Cuol: 'What is your father's name?'

I: 'My father's name is also Pritchard.'

Cuol: 'No, that cannot be true, you cannot have the same name as your father.'

I: 'It is the name of my lineage. What is the name of your lineage?'

Cuol: 'Do you want to know the name of my lineage?'

I: 'Yes.'

Cuol: 'What will you do with it if I tell you? Will you take it to your country?'

I: 'I don't want to do anything with it. I just want to know it since I am living at your camp.'

Cuol: 'Oh well, we are Lou.'

I: 'I did not ask you the name of your tribe. I know that. I am asking you the name of your lineage.'

Coul: 'Why do you want to know the name of my lineage?'

I: 'I don't want to know it.'

Cuol: 'Then why do you ask me for it? Give me some tobacco.'

I defy the most patient ethnologist to make headway against this kind of opposition [concluded Evans-Pritchard].

Interviewees are people with considerable potential for sabotaging the attempt to research them. Where, as in the case of anthropology or repeated interviewing in sociology, the research cannot proceed without a relationship of mutual trust being established between interviewer and interviewee the prospects are particularly dismal. This inevitably changes the interviewer/anthropologist's attitude to the people he/she is studying. A poignant example is the incident related in Elenore Smith Bowen's[20] *Return to Laughter* when the anthropologist witnesses one of her most trusted informants dying in childbirth (1956, p.163):

I stood over Amara. She tried to smile at me. She was very ill. I was convinced these women could not help her. She would die. She was my friend but my epitaph for her would be impersonal observations scribbled in my notebook, her memory preserved in an anthropologist's file: 'Death (in childbirth)/Cause: witchcraft/Case of Amara.' A lecture from the past reproached me: 'The anthropologist cannot, like the chemist or biologist, arrange controlled experiments. Like the astronomer, his mere presence produces changes in the data he is trying to observe. He himself is a disturbing influence which he must endeavour to keep to the minimum. His claim to science must therefore rest on a meticulous accuracy of observations and on a cool, objective approach to his data.'

A cool, objective approach to Amara's death?

One can, perhaps, be cool when dealing with questionnaires or when interviewing strangers. But what is one to do when one can collect one's data only by forming personal friendships? It is hard enough to think of a friend as a case history. Was I to stand aloof, observing the course of events?

Professional hesitation meant that Bowen might never see the ceremonies connected with death in childbirth. But, on the other hand, she would see her friend die. Bowen's difficult decision to plead with Amara's kin and the midwives in charge of her case to allow her access to Western medicine did not pay off and Amara did eventually die.

An anthropologist has to 'get inside the culture'; participant observation means 'that . . . the observer participates in the daily life of the people under study, either openly in the role of researcher or covertly in some disguised role' (Becker and Geer, 1957, p.28). A feminist interviewing women is by definition both 'inside' the culture and participating in that which she is observing. However, in these respects the behaviour of a feminist interviewer/researcher is not extraordinary. Although (Stanley and Wise, 1979, pp.359–61)

Descriptions of the research process in the social sciences often suggest that the motivation for carrying out sub-

Ann Oakley

stantive work lies in theoretical concerns ... the research process appears a very orderly and coherent process indeed..... The personal tends to be carefully removed from public statements; these are full of rational argument [and] careful discussion of academic points. [It can equally easily be seen that] all research is 'grounded', because no researcher can separate herself from personhood and thus from deriving second order constructs from experience.

A feminist methodology of social science requires that this rationale of research be described and discussed not only in feminist research but in social science research in general. It requires, further, that the mythology of 'hygienic' research with its accompanying mystification of the researcher and the researched as objective instruments of data production be replaced by the recognition that personal involvement is more than dangerous bias — it is the condition under which people come to know each other and to admit others into their lives.

Notes

1 I am not dealing with others, such as self-administered questionnaires, here since not quite the same framework applies.
2 For Galtung (1967, p.138) the appropriate metaphor is a thermometer.
3 Most interviewers are, of course, female.
4 Many 'respondents' are, of course, female.
5 See Hyman *et al.* (1955).
6 This label suggests that the interviewer's role is to get the interviewee to 'inform' (somewhat against his/her will) on closely guarded and dangerous secrets.
7 Benney and Hughes (1970) discuss interviewing in terms of the dual conventions or 'fictions' of equality and comparability.
8 Moser (1958, p.185) says, 'since most interviewers are women I shall refer to them throughout as of the female sex.'
9 I attended six of the births.
10 What I have to say about my experience of interviewing relates to my own experience and not that of my research assistant.
11 I am grateful to the Social Science Research Council for funding the research and to Bedford College, London University, for administering it.

12   The interviews were fully transcribed and the analysis then done from the transcripts.
13   The women all had their babies at the same London maternity hospital.
14   I had, of course, made it clear to the women I was interviewing that I had no medical training, but as I have argued elsewhere (Oakley, 1981b) mothers do not see medical experts as the only legitimate possessors of knowledge about motherhood.
15   It is, however, an important part of the Rapoports' definition of 'interactive research' that psychoanalytic principles should be applied in analysing processes of 'transference'and 'counter-transference' in the interviewer–interviewee relationship.
16   See Mitchell and Oakley (1976) and Oakley (1981a) on the idea of sisterhood.
17   See Smith (1979).
18   Both these were telephone contacts only. See Oakley (1980), chapter 4, for more on the research methods used.
19   Hobson observes that her approach to interviewing women yielded no refusals to co-operate.
20   Elenore Smith Bowen is a pseudonym for a well-known anthropologist.

References

Becker, H.S. and Geer, B. (1957), 'Participant Observation and Interviewing: A Comparison? *Human Organisation*, vol. XVI, pp.28-32.

Bell, C. and Encel, S. (eds) (1978), *Inside the Whale*, Pergamon Press, Oxford.

Bell, C. and Encel, S. (1978) 'Introduction' to Bell and Encel (eds), *Inside the Whale*, Pergamon Press, Oxford.

Bell, C. and Newby, H. (1977), *Doing Sociological Research*, Allen & Unwin, London.

Benney, M. and Hughes, E.C. (1970), 'Of Sociology and the Interview' in N.K. Denzin (ed.), *Sociological Methods: A Source Book*, Butterworth, London.

Bernard, J. (1975), *Women, Wives, Mothers*, Aldine, Chicago.

Bowen, E.S. (1956), *Return to Laughter*, Gollancz, London.

Corbin, M. (1971), 'Appendix 3' in J.M. and R.E. Pahl, *Managers and their Wives*, Allen Lane, London.

Denzin, N.K. (1970) (ed.), *Sociological Methods: A Source Book*, Butterworth, London.

Denzin, N.K. (1970) 'Introduction: Part V' in N.K. Denzin (ed.), *Sociological Methods: A Source Book*, Butterworth, London.

Dexter, L.A. (1956), 'Role Relationships and Conceptions of Neutrality in Interviewing', *American Journal of Sociology*, vol. LX14, p.153-7.

Evans-Pritchard, E.E. (1940), *The Nuer*, Oxford University Press, London.

Fransella, F. and Frost, K. (1977), *On Being a Woman*, Tavistock, London.

Galtung, J. (1967), *Theory and Methods of Social Research*, Allen & Unwin, London.

Goode, W.J. and Hatt, P.K. (1952), *Methods in Social Research*, McGraw Hill, New York.

Griffiths, D. and Saraga, E. (1979), 'Sex Differences and Cognitive Abilities: A Sterile Field of Enquiry' in O. Hartnett *et al.* (eds), *Sex Role Stereotyping*, Tavistock, London.

Hartnett, O., Boden, G. and Fuller, M. (eds) (1979) *Sex-Role Stereotyping*, Tavistock, London.

Hobson, D. (1978), 'Housewives: Isolation as Oppression' in Women's Studies Group, Centre for Contemporary Cultural Studies, *Women Take Issue*, Hutchinson, London.

Hochschild, A.R. (1975), 'The Sociology of Feeling and Emotion: Selected Possibilities' in M. Millman and R.M. Kanter (eds), *Another Voice: Feminist Perspectives on Social Life and Social Science*, Anchor Books, New York.

Hyman, H.H. *et al.* (1955), *Interviewing in Social Research*, University of Chicago Press.

Kahn, R.L. and Cannell, L.F. (1957), *The Dynamics of Interviewing*, John Wiley, New York.

Laslett, B. and Rapoport, R. (1975), 'Collaborative Interviewing and Interactive Research', *Journal of Marriage and the Family*, November, pp.968–77.

Mamak, A.F. (1978), *Nationalism, Race-Class Consciousness and Social Research on Bougainville Island, Papua, New Guinea*, in C. Bell and S. Encel (eds), *Inside the Whale*, Pergamon Press, Oxford.

Miller, J.B. (1976), *Toward a New Psychology of Women*, Beacon Press, Boston.

Mitchell, J. and Oakley A. (1976), 'Introduction' in J. Mitchell and A. Oakley (eds), *The Rights and Wrongs of Women*, Penguin, Harmondsworth.

Moser, C.A. (1958), *Survey Methods in Social Investigation*, Heinemann, London.

Oakley, A. (1972), *Sex, Gender and Society*, Maurice Temple Smith, London.

Oakley. A. (1974), *The Sociology of Housework*, Martin Robertson, London.

Oakley, A. (1979), *Becoming a Mother*, Martin Robertson, Oxford.

Oakley, A. (1980), *Women Confined: Towards a Sociology of Childbirth*, Martin Robertson, Oxford.

Oakley, A. (1981a), *Subject Women*, Martin Robertson, Oxford.

Oakley, A. (1981b), 'Normal Motherhood: An Exercise in Self-Control', in B. Hutter and G. Williams (eds), *Controlling Women*, Croom Helm, London.

Paul, B. (1954), 'Interview Techniques and Field Relationships' in A.C. Kroeber (ed.), *Anthropology Today,* University of Chicago Press.

Rapoport, R. and Rapoport, R. (1976), *Dual Career Families Reexamined,* Martin Robertson, London.

Richardson, S.A. *et al.* (1965), *Interviewing: its Forms and Functions,* Basic Books, New York.

Rose, A.M. (1945), 'A Research Note on Experimentation in Interviewing', *American Journal of Sociology,* vol. 51 pp.143-4.

Sayers, J. (1979), *On the Description of Psychological Sex Differences* in O. Hartnett *et al.* (eds), *Sex Role Stereotyping,* Tavistock, London.

Selltiz, C., Jahoda, M., Deutsch, M. and Cook, S.W. (1965), *Research Methods in Social Relations,* Methuen, London.

Shipman, M.D. (1972), *The Limitations of Social Research,* Longman, London.

Sjoberg, G. and Nett, R. (1968), *A Methodology for Social Research,* Harper & Row, New York.

Smith, D.E. (1979), 'A Sociology for Women' in J.A. Sherman and E.T. Beck (eds), *The Prism of Sex,* University of Wisconsin Press, Madison.

Stacey, M. (1969), *Methods of Social Research,* Pergamon, Oxford.

Stanley, L. and Wise, S. (1979), 'Feminist Research, Feminist Consciousness and Experiences of Sexism', *Women's Studies International Quarterly,* vol. 2, no. 3, pp.359-79.

Zweig, F. (1949), *Labour, Life and Poverty,* Gollancz, London.

3

Reminiscences of fieldwork among the Sikhs[1]

Joyce Pettigrew

Though I consider that anthropology is a science, we all know that both in the collecting and in the interpreting of our data, social and personal interests are deeply involved. Hence the subject itself requires that we understand something of the situations in which particular practitioners worked and wrote. In examining myself, I examine the subject (Max Gluckman, *Order and Rebellion in Tribal Africa*, 1963, pp.vii–viii).

This chapter describes the fieldwork difficulties faced by a young female anthropologist working among landowning Sikhs in the Punjab and the effects of sex and kinship ties on the research situation. Pettigrew's research as such — on the role played by rural factions in building up the power of state-level political leaders — was not concerned with sexual divisions, but working as a woman in this situation raised important issues of access to data and power relationships, which she discusses in detail. Finally, Pettigrew analyses her choice of research topic and suggests reasons for her choice at that time of a study of the powerful rather than the powerless.

It has been noted that 'the study of culture and society has advanced to the point where we are more aware of the theoretical importance, actual or conceivable of the data we are losing' (Sturtevant, 1967, p.355). The statement relates to the disappearance of cultural variations. Equally it might be regarded as a realistic commentary on what is a typical research situation for an anthropologist, where much of the information he/she could potentially collect is, in fact, out of reach due to the place and position she or he occupies in the society she or he studies. Evans-Pritchard (1964) makes a number of references as to how this can result in the gathering of either inaccurate or insufficient information. It is, however, notably Cicourel (1964)[2] and Freilich (1970)[3] who have argued the importance of explaining the set of circumstances and conditions that favourably or unfavourably influence data collection. Freilich believes that 'if field experiences are shared many common errors could be avoided.' (p.31) Berreman (1962) also regrets the absence of information 'on the practical problems of carrying out fieldwork.' (p.4)[4]

In this chapter I give a picture of my own research situation among landowning Sikhs (Jats) during a first fieldwork trip to the Punjab in the years 1965–7 and which later resulted in the publication of *Robber Noblemen* (Pettigrew, 1975). My fieldwork area was part of a rich farming region some fifteen miles east and south of one of the Punjab's major cities — Ludhiana. I had gone to the Punjab when the war between Pakistan and India had just begun. At that time it seemed impossible to work in an area where one was not known and since I had married into a Jat family belonging to Ludhiana district I went to stay with those relatives who held their ancestral land there. My own fieldwork situation was to become particularly affected by my residence with them. But this aside, the events I describe below testify to the existence of an actual situation of which any young woman will have to take account as well as operate in should she choose to work alone in the Punjab, east or west, or in the Middle East. The nature of Jat society in the rural areas thirteen years ago, especially its attitudes towards women, was a factor significantly influencing the nature and course of my social interactions during fieldwork. But conditions throughout the area from Istanbul eastwards, as reported by Fernea and Bezirgan (1976) and Papanek (1964) would appear to indicate this would be a significant variable influencing the course of fieldwork for any woman.

In the rural Punjab, a woman is significant as a mother of sons whom she hopes to make powerful and influential, and as a sister whom her brothers want to marry into a family that will raise their status. Women are usually secluded and conduct their life separately from men. Customarily they have not been expected to talk to men except on certain prescribed occasions. In villages if they do not practise actual physical *purdah* (for information on *purdah* see Papanek, (1973) and Jacobson (1976)) they remain indoors most of the time, and when they do go out they do so with their head covered and eyes lowered. The reputation of the family depends on the behaviour and conduct of its women. Thus, especially when women have to travel alone, a certain amount of nervousness is visible in their behaviour. If a man stops a young woman on the road to ask her the way, a not uncommon reply is 'Have you no sister or mother to ask the way from?' For one consequence of the separation between the sexes is that a young woman seen talking to a man is invariably suspected of having a sexual relationship with him. That this conclusion is reached often when the two people are not in any such relation is because the only place of contact between men and women is the bed. They do not eat together, do not sit and talk together and only on rare occasions go out together. To be seen with a man, therefore, damages a woman's reputation. Reputation depends less on what one actually does than on what those around think one to be doing and what is subsequently talked about one. Where one goes, and with whom one goes in public are the subject of much comment, and the content of that comment constitutes one's reputation. A woman shares in the reputation of the man with whom she is seen. Two cardinal rules for a woman, therefore, are that she should not go 'here and there', and that she should not be seen with a person whose reputation is already bad.

A third rule for a woman is that she should not go out alone. There are now few actual instances of rape and abduction, but a widespread fear of rape and abduction persists. With the solitary woman any man feels free to strike up a conversation, the object being to boast later to his friends and to give an impression to them, as to all around, that he is acquainted with her. And again, because of the traditional separation of the sexes, and because the sole legitimate access to women is through marriage, for a man to talk to a woman thus is for him in the nature of an adventure. Travelling around alone for a woman can thus be dangerous since it brings men to look upon her in a certain way. It is an encouragement and an invitation for any man who is daring enough, and hence it brings a stigma on to the woman. It is, in fact, in many instances, the prelude to actual danger. Perhaps the hazard is still greater for a European woman because she is fair-skinned and because her reputation in Muslim and Sikh society is that she can be easily seduced.

This was an aspect of the social situation during my fieldwork that intimately affected both my work and myself. I was made aware of it through my own experiences and unreservedly by the attitudes of family members. These rules governing a woman's meetings and movements were not at all practical for me to follow. My research concentrated on a political problem — that of the role played by rural factions in building up the power of state-level political leaders, and I was endeavouring to understand why factions, as a form of organisation, were preventing the centralisation of political power in the state. This project involved innumerable and sustained contacts with political leaders and their supporters in local areas. Both these categories had bad reputations. The society's attitude towards me was that if I was not of bad character myself, then why did I need to have contact with bad persons? No one credited me with maintaining many of these relationships solely for utilitarian purposes. And, if I ignored a snide remark instead of getting the situation more dramatically remedied, it was condemned as acquiescence, synonymous with ignoring 'insult'; ignoring those who were doing 'harm to one's name'. One had to forget one's own cultural precept that indifference was not tolerance and to display at once and for all to see, one's opposition, in order to maintain one's respect.

The operating principles of rural society were those of re-ciprocity and patronage and these affected my fieldwork. A specific kind of interpersonal relationship was set up between those who asked for, and those who granted, requests. To give was to do favour to, and when favours were accepted a return was expected, at a moment appropriate to the donor and on a basis of what that party wanted to have and receive, and not on the basis of what one was capable of giving. That, combined with the fact that Jat Sikhs enjoyed women — and that not being a permanent operating part of the system one's position was such that one could not offer any concrete ad-vantages — produced at times a set of circumstances that were very difficult to control.

In the account of my fieldwork experience that follows, it will be evident that there was little integration in the roles I occupied as a young woman anthropologist from Europe and the wife of a Jat. The conflict between those roles emerged most in the rural areas when my behaviour and activities were decided by my affinal ties and my links with a particular family. This was to a lesser extent the case when meeting administrative officials in the state capital of Chandigarh. These I met in my individual capacity as an anthropologist and they were interested in the nature of my work. That I was the wife of a Jat remained only a topic of casual, happy conversation and curiosity.

The family into which I had married had owned thousands of acres of land in what is now Malawi. Although they had lost it due to what may be termed political caprice in the very same year in which my fieldwork began, village society in Punjab still regarded me as a landlord's wife. The family's inherited land was in any case still cultivated by a formidable *Daddiji* (paternal grandmother) while *Mamaji* (mother's brother) was not only the Sirdar of his village but controlled through debt relationships the surrounding five villages. *Mamaji*'s sole surviving heir had married the only sister of six brothers who headed one of the area's two factions and who were powerful and feared. They cultivated an acreage of land that was extremely high for District Ludhiana — 245 acres — as well as owning 400 acres in Uttar Pradesh. To them *Mamaji's* family, in which I stayed, were very close and the relationship established by marriage was used in many matters both major and minor. I was particularly close to the then head of the family since my husband, as a child, used to play with him and his brothers when he came back to the village from his boarding school in the hills. My own affinal connection hence meant that I had greater access to the participants in one of the two factions concerned. However, I doubt if gathering most of my information from one faction to the exclusion of the other was solely a product of that alone. Inevitably, without the existence of any such tie, I could not have been trusted equally by both factions had I shifted to and fro simply for purposes of collecting information.

The family's network of relationships was decidedly my own, whether I liked it or not, and because of my affinal connection, certain persons were not accessible to me. It prevented me, for example, from meeting two prominent members of the faction opposing my relatives. I could not meet the first for reasons of personal safety: my affines felt that the person concerned would have regarded it as his duty to arrange to dishonour me in some way. I had arranged three times to meet the other man — an MLA (Member of the Legislative Assembly) — one of these meetings being in a *gurudwara* (Sikh temple) — but on none of these occasions did he turn up. I later learned that he suspected I was leading him into a trap to have him murdered. Due to such factors, my documentation of the activities of one faction was richer.[5] However, I was able to stay in the house of an important member of the opposing faction, making the excuse that his was the only good house available in which to live. Moreover, all my information was not solely gained from members of factions themselves. Luckily, I also managed to collect data from local lawyers in the District Courts at Ludhiana and Patiala, press correspondents, *pancayat* (village council) officers and officers of the Criminal Investigation Department, and from the judgments given in court cases in which members of factions were involved. When I was collecting information on faction leaders at state level, my family relationships were again of use to me, though often in an obscure fashion. To give one example: in March 1966 I had been staying with the then Registrar of Punjabi University, whose son had been at school with my husband's younger brother. This was the basis of my introduction to the family. During my stay there, a relative of a former Chief Minister of the Punjab visited the Registrar whom he much admired. Noticing that I was on very friendly terms with the Registrar and his family, he offered his help to me at the end of his stay, should I ever need it. When I visited his home later he showed me a number of documents which enabled me to substantiate as fact a number of statements made by certain political leaders at state level regarding their political alignments. Merely being in certain homes gave one some credibility. For example, being seen to stay in a Chief Justice's house when he was visited by the Public Prosecutor of the district in which one worked certainly encouraged the latter to trust one and be a bit more malleable over access to court records.

Much of the information I gathered had this quality of being apparently accidentally obtained. However, especially in my relationship with the civil and police administration, members of the legislature and leaders of political parties, I did owe much to the presence of my husband for six months. He was able to define my position unequivocally as the wife of a Jat in some instances and the wife of a Sikh in others and, where necessary, the wife of a Punjabi. Moreover, it was precisely when my husband was there that I was entitled to move around socially. It was then that I obtained access to persons to whom otherwise I would have found difficulty in relating myself. Having an affinal link in this particular set of circumstances, therefore, put me in the position of being able to form an acquaintanceship with key persons in the social surroundings of an exclusive club or at a private party in their home. When I later wanted to contact them for certain pieces of information, it was much easier to re-establish relationships.

Inevitably any fieldworker can only know of what is going on around him or her, what she or he can fortunately observe and only so much as people are willing to yield up to him or her. In a society where the movement of women outside their houses is always restricted and supervised, the demands and needs of one's work to move around and to talk freely to innumerable people, but chiefly men, contradict social expectancies and contradict the status in which the society places the wife of a Jat. There can be only one interpretation placed on the activities of a woman who does not seclude herself and who insists, as the society sees it, on talking to men. My relatives intermittently helped in overcoming the difficulties of this actual situation by accompanying me whenever they could and enabling me thus to move around more than I could otherwise have done without danger.

From my closeted position I certainly often queried whether an objective danger awaited me in those houses into which I was forewarned by my relatives not to stray, or on a *kaccha* (dirt) road connecting a village to the main metalled road, if I walked along it at dusk, or whether this was merely the product of how I was being conditioned to think. Perhaps the danger was actual; and the rules were applied to me to protect my own honour and for my own respect and well-being. I can scarcely forget how one evening after dark, in one of the small towns ridden by factional rivalry, when I had to move a short distance from the truck union of one of the factions to the house in which I was staying overnight. I was immediately provided with an encircling body of four armed men, three of them my affines. I also remember how my husband and I spent a perfectly comfortable week together in the house of a member of the opposing faction. We were always treated respectfully. But when my husband went away and I had to remain there without him, the situation altered.

Protectors were needed and, as a result, the bulk of my information on local area factionalism was collected, and some of my most satisfactory information gathered, in conditions when I was under such protection. Usually this was family protection or protection arranged by the family. I always regretted, however, that I could participate in so few of the male drinking parties and hear personally some of the useful gossip that seemed to be exchanged on those occasions. But there were occasions when, thanks to my affines, I could freely let hours pass by indulging my curiosity. Then since I was a young woman of an unusual social type for them this certainly went in my favour. I doubt if some of the characters participating in the factionalism would have spent so much time talking to a man!

Jats have in their minds certain stereotypes about their

women, namely that they were weak, helpless and stupid. They applied them to me also and it would seem that sometimes I benefited from being so regarded. They always assumed that I could not pick up the allusions they would freely scatter when drunk or have the strength to follow them up afterwards. However, my right to enquire, watch and observe freely always had to be guaranteed by someone influential or respected. The situation I was placed in without such protection often startlingly revealed to me the nature of those whom I had been thinking to be epitomes of civic virtue. And it was in such situations, when I was defenceless, that I could perceive the truth of certain facts which I had been given about the behaviour of certain persons and about which I had been previously always somewhat incredulous. Such behaviour, as well as confirming reports of how a man had behaved at particular moments in time in the past to others who were similarly without protection, also exhibited clues which I could later check in a more substantial way, to gain information about his activities in the present.

The practical difficulties any young woman will face in gathering information in this type of society irrespective of any affinal connexion she may have are evident. If she moves freely, the consequent lack of respect likely to be felt for her acting thus will prevent her from getting into the inside of many matters. If she does not pursue her information, the quality of her work will be similarly affected through lack of the appropriate data on many topics. That is her dilemma. This was partially offset and overcome in my own case by my being married into the community: some of my affines were able to accompany me on certain occasions and by their physical presence they played a significant role in my information collecting. But any young woman working in this or a similar type of society may expect to have her search for data constantly delayed by the tension in her mind stemming from a situation where the integrity of herself and her work are in contradiction and from the problem: how much of 'self' should be sacrificed for the sake of data? In my own case the presence of affines helped by reducing the number of occasions on which I was placed in this situation and experienced this contradiction.

Being a member of a Jat family provided me with help, not only in carrying out my fieldwork on a day-to-day basis, but also quickened my assimilation to Jat society. As part of a Jat family, I had a role, a position and a status assigned to me from the beginning of my fieldwork. Instant socialisation was expected of me. I had been accepted into the family as a young wife, so I was expected to follow a wife's pattern of behaviour, and conform also to the rules of rural Jat society. Being a member of a family at once placed me within a wide range of relationships in the society too, all of which, when I did not behave as a Jat woman, were bent on teaching me how. I had to quickly give up any sort of resistance to covering my head, partially veiling my face, covering the top parts of my arms and so forth. If I had failed to comply with these customs a lack of sympathy certainly would have developed on the part of those among whom I lived.[6] They found it very difficult to appreciate that I had come to Punjab for an educational purpose. No one could understand why a young woman married to a tall, handsome Jat could leave him and her home to make a study thousands of miles away from both.

The family's intention in forcing me to observe certain rules was that I (and they) might be well regarded in the wider society. Doing so shielded me — if only in the small circle of those known — from being the victim of the rationalisation that I was 'a loose woman'. I had moved into a society that felt its superiority in all spheres except the technological. And it was a society that had formed an advance opinion of me, as a western woman, before I had entered it; and which was only prepared to alter that opinion if I accepted and conformed to its own pattern of family relationships. That I became immediately and suddenly open to a new manner of socialisation was, however, specifically because I was a member of a family. In my capacity as a young wife the family had a claim on me in terms of behaviour, while I had an access by right to them. For me all the families I met were not just 'families of the fieldwork area', but they were families connected to my own in various ways. How they regarded me was not only important to me because I knew that if I were highly esteemed I would get more co-operation, but I also saw my-

self, as indeed they saw me, as part of a set of relationships
that would be permanent.

My socialisation to the new way of life was accomplished
by all these families repeating the same set of injunctions with
respect to my behaviour. One aspect of my socialisation for
me as a woman consisted of learning to accept that I could
not go out except when it was arranged. On the occasions when
I did go out I soon became terrified of meeting a man's gaze
and, worse still, of letting a smile slip on to my face while
talking to men. Affines, therefore, always sought to control
my movements. Thus on days when my interpreter or other
chaperone failed to turn up I could rarely get out of the house.
And during the 1967 general elections, there was a quarrel
within the family about whether I should be allowed to go into one of the election cars, one female family member going
red in the face and stamping her feet determinedly with the
words 'saadi apni' ('she's our very own'). On this occasion it
was only my husband's decision to postpone his departure
for Delhi and to accompany me until the elections were over
that gave me the freedom to travel and observe election activities in the local area.

A second aspect of my socialisation in the rural areas at
that time was that I had to train myself not to talk to men.
Hence I could not approach them with questions. Adherence
to the rules of separation was very difficult. The only time
the men spent with the women was in bed. In the evenings
when they returned home from the fields or the market they
ate separately, talking and chatting among themselves. They
did so in comfortable armchairs with tables in front of them,
indoors, and the women sat outside around the cooking square,
on low stools (*püris*), bending over their food which was eaten
off circular trays (*thals*) and not tables. The men were served
first by the women. Indeed, a woman had no right to go into
the men's room at all; she had no place there. I, for example,
could not, and very rarely did, speak to the head of the household; and my requests, even for medicine, I remember, would
do a circle of his eldest daughter, his wife and his sons, before
reaching him. In this situation for me to think of going into
the men's room to ask questions on matters that interested
me was almost a revolutionary idea. When my husband was

there he would report back on what had been said. But, if he was not, the fact that I could not speak freely to the head of the household resulted in an undoubted loss of information. He could have been a key informant on the happenings of the area, financially controlling as he did the neighbouring villages and maintaining as he did an intimate relationship with local officials and the head of one of the factions. Sometimes I sought permission to go and ask questions and, on occasions, when my request was taken notice of and granted, I dreaded it for hours beforehand. Finally, over my *daal* (lentils) and *chapattis* (flat wheat cakes), I would prepare myself to make the effort to cross the stretch of room between the door and the place where the men sat with what would appear as confidence and grace. Men made themselves special by this separation. Although all my husband's young cousins who had BA degrees silently felt resentful at this, publicly they and I would fall in with the habit of respecting this pattern of avoidance.

The hardest part of fieldwork, then, was to concern myself solely with my own motivations in the face of constant evaluation according to different rules and standards by those around me. I, like the other young women in the family, found it difficult not to feel inferior and shy in the presence of men and in some instances this affected the pace of my fieldwork. I had to remind myself continually that I was primarily an anthropologist. The effect of Jat society on me as mediated through the relationships formed by marriage, the sort of self it was moulding, was one building up inhibition after inhibition, and this enormously influenced my ability and willingness to collect data. I doubt if my sensitivity would have been so crippling had I not been part of a Jat family, in close connection also with the community and, therefore, under pressure to pay deference to its customs. My membership of a Jat family undoubtedly made me more conscious of the society's rules both when I was disobeying and obeying them. It did so from a viewpoint other than that of an interest in collecting information. My response to these rules was set not only in a pragmatic context — to obtain the information I needed — but also, in addition, was felt as an obligation.

The effects of this type of socialisation on the personality of any woman coming from an urban, industrialised society will be such as to affect her attitudes towards, and ultimately her capacities to do, her fieldwork. Psychological effects are especially evident on a first field trip. In my own case my receptiveness to the society's rulings, views and way of life, in the form of burning hate or dutiful obedience, was merely intensified because I was related to it by marriage.

For example, I hated rural Jat society's attitudes to feminine beauty. Beauty was always to be hidden; for inevitably it would be the cause of some destruction. A beautiful woman suffered more, her family being apprehensive of a situation in which she would place their honour in danger by attracting covetous eyes. As Camus noted, but with respect to nations not women, 'The countries which harbour beauty are the most difficult to defend — one would like so much to spare them.' And the same could be said for young Jat women, fair-skinned and slender as many of them were. I hated the violence done to the minds and bodies of my husband's young cousins by seclusion, hidden behind the walls of the house, behind a *dupatta* (the long scarf which covers the shoulder and upper part of a woman's body and, in rural areas, also her head and face). Daily I watched the destruction of my sister-in-law's beauty — her ballerina's face, and her walk envisioning the flight of a swallow. This happening became for me more than a momentary aggravation, set as it was in a landscape of serenity and romance. It was something for which to mourn. But by all others in the family and the village it passed unnoticed. And her opposite — fat, greasy, old and ugly — hovered over the household, ordering and intruding into everything. I felt this to be wrong. Perhaps I experienced the cruelty done to the younger members of the family as a personal wound because I myself was then young, and I felt the way of life was making me ugly too. The continuous bending over pumps countless times in the day, sitting on *püris* and bending over food, had destroyed my posture. Mosquito bites had scarred my arms and feet. And, because we did not go out much and did not get any exercise, we were unable to look after our bodies and had inevitably got fat.

Throughout this period I had been eating my food out in the open around the fire with the women, dressing as they did also, practically, in a flowing *kameez* (shirt), and wide *salwar* (loose trousers), sleeping out at night on a *charpoy* (string bed) under a dark sky and, in the morning, rising at five and saying Sikh prayers to the rhythmic swish of water over my body. This was enjoyment rather than difficulty. But I was shocked by some of my seemingly unconscious responses to typical village situations. The remembrance of one of these particularly remains very much alive. Once, on a very hot day, at noon, I was eating lunch in the men's room, cool at last, comfortable in a chair and free of my *dupatta*. Suddenly there was the noise of *Mamaji* arriving back, quite unexpectedly earlier than usual. I rushed out of the room leaving both food and *dupatta* behind, but unfortunately not quickly enough. I collided with him at the door and felt ashamed that I had been discovered sitting in a place where I was not supposed to be and, in addition, with my head uncovered. It was if I had been caught while committing a crime. And a visit to Ludhiana after many uninterrupted weeks of village life crystallised my situation. I felt a typical village woman emerging out of *purdah* and not knowing how to cope.[7] The experience was harsh. My field-work was becoming what in effect was their life — a wanton destruction of beauty, physically by disfigurement, emotionally by deprivation. I realised that I would have to check the sort of development that was making it difficult for me to meet and talk with people as well as travel on my own. I would have to learn anew how to do all these things. The habit of avoiding men was not a custom strictly practised outside the village, nor was that of respectful silence before men and elders. In the village it had seemed as if I had lost the facility to express myself through feeling that I had to conform to a system in which shyness in a woman was a value. Had I not had the opportunity to go on holiday at this juncture, I would never have been able to retain the 'self' that had gone to Punjab not to become *Jatti*,[8] but to do anthropological fieldwork.[9] A chance visit of my husband's *sakhi bra* (literally, true brother; brother in faith and trust) gave me the chance to travel without family suspicion to a hill station, to Delhi, and to Chandigarh, the state capital.

In Delhi, particularly, I felt like a piece of hewn wood. And I was totally unprepared for the sense of distance I would feel from people of my own culture. I was envious of the

European women I saw, with their short hair and their legs freely showing, their gay lipsticks and chic clothes. These few glimpses reminded me that I too had been part of their world. This temporarily helped by giving me a different reference point: a series of pictorial images other than fields, veiled faces, murders and *charpoys*. But equally, I felt a sense of desperation and I conceived it impossible that I would ever return to Europe.

My work in the rural areas had given me a preoccupation with being a Jat woman rather than an anthropologist, and hence was in the process of leading me into steadily increasing seclusion both from my own culture and from my discipline. My stay in Chandigarh, during which my husband's friend gave me contacts in the administration, was helpful, in that it meant I had to learn again how to talk to reasonably sophisticated men without being shy. My holiday was turned into a stay of three months which advanced my research still further. It is interesting to note how a decision taken at the time for reasons of personal stress aided my work.[10] For it was as a result of my stay in the state capital and the information I gathered there that I was able to appreciate the extent to which the factionalism of the local area in which I worked was related to the political developments at state level and the degree to which it was known throughout the Punjab. Factions were statewide units.

When I returned to the village, it was with a confidence that my affines could not drown my aims though I still remained acutely sensitive as to what was expected from me. I would alternate erratically between extreme subservience to their wishes that I stay indoors, or, under pressure and a feeling of frustration of what still had to be done, would be far too adventurous and make plans to accomplish my work on my own. I then rebelled, albeit uncomfortably, against instructions not to move around. This, indeed, was to remain the only sphere in which contradiction lay between the family of which I was a part and myself. Otherwise, during my two years in the field, my response to situations imperceptibly became more and more those of the local inhabitants. In a given situation, therefore, I did not feel in a position to judge whether the local response was the most effective or not.

In some respects I felt a complete *Jatti*. That I did feel in this way was because the set of ties I had been using fairly persistently were ties from one particular section of the family: its landowning section. My involvement was sustained by them and, during my first fieldwork visit, I did not feel free to form a relationship with the Punjab of my own choosing.

The principal theoretical considerations why 'anthropologists anonymous' should attempt an analysis of their fieldwork experiences are that their data is gathered through interaction, as persons with other persons. Necessarily, therefore, one has to focus on the type of relationships one develops in the area where one works. It is also essential to recognise, and subsequently develop, the implications of that realisation, that not all anthropologists are in a position to gather the information they want. I have indicated my own limitations in the rural Punjab. I also remember an occasion when one anthropologist who was working among the Sikh Jats mentioned his indebtedness to his Punjabi wife without whom, he claims, he would have had difficulty discovering matters of importance. Often the anthropological role as such is inadequate for collecting certain types of information. I felt conscious of this in a different way when doing my second piece of research on the Jat immigrant community in England. On one occasion when meeting a Special Branch Officer I felt both helpless and despondent that the detailed information that he possessed was of the type I needed and that it was being collected more effectively by a non-anthropologist. Both these factors may mean that some of the theoretical considerations we draw are based on unsatisfactory evidence. I have, however, presented the above extended account of my fieldwork experiences for another more important reason.

My connection with the community was a permanent one. This being so, the time dimension to my relationships was correspondingly different from that of a fieldworker who occupies the role of a stranger within the community and who, therefore, has greater freedom in breaking as well as in renewing his ties with them. Rural Jat society and its attitudes had a deep impact on me and I feel that in writing this very personal document I have not merely catalogued my own miseries and joys over a period of two years but also spoken from a woman's standpoint of the organisation of a particular society and culture. All fieldworkers should feel justified in exploring their experiences and encounters in the field for, to the extent to which they have moved in rhythm with, touched the spontaneity of, and been near to and free with those among whom they lived, they have experienced the entry of another culture and another set of values into their own being. Thus, while writing about one's own field experiences may seem an extraordinary personal exposé, what is more significant is that it is also a discovery and revelation of the nature of the society in which one lived from one particular stance. To this I now return.

The variables involved in each research situation are different. In this chapter, I have sought to present and examine the nature of the two most important variables affecting my own fieldwork conditions in the Punjab — that of being a young western woman anthropologist, and of being married to a Jat. On the surface, one problem appears to be whether the nature of my fieldwork conditions, as outlined here, would evidence that a woman is not suited to gather information in that class of societies whose pattern of social organisation is influenced by the notion of *purdah*. It could be said that the nature of the resocialisation demanded of a woman in such a society means that she gathers so little of the data she knows to be potentially available.[11] She has to be protected to do her work at all. And this would be especially true of a woman who is, in addition, not related to a family in the fieldwork area, and who is without influential and trustworthy friends.

My own experiences, related to my structural position in the household as a young, newly married woman, could lead me to conclude that it is highly unrealistic for other women in a similar position to select such societies for study on their own. But it has to be kept in mind that the problems covered by my research involved intensive contact with men. Minimal contact would have been necessary had I examined the relationships between various categories of women within the property group, while beyond the household, young mothers and the under-fives comprised a significant section of the under-privileged in any Punjabi village, particularly from the viewpoint of health care. Any problem relating to mother and child health in rural communities could have been selected and it is doubtful if the difficulties indicated in this chapter would have been encountered. It seems strange to me now that although I and all the young daughters-in-law were in a similar learning situation and actually sharing many of the same experiences and capable of sharing still more, yet my participation in their lives and problems did not direct me to analyse their social condition. Thus though I had access to the sphere of pain so frequently the domain of the young daughter-in-law in a rural Punjabi household, I neglected its description and explanation and consigned it to my private diary. I, as an anthropologist, thought of a man's unmarried sisters and daughters in exactly the same way as he himself did, namely as a means to make profitable links with other property groups.

The explanation for my attitudes does not lie in my own individual self but in anthropology as it was then. When I first went out to the field, anthropologists were supposed to report customs without the addition to their account of any evaluative element. Value-commitments, whatever their nature, rarely determined the foci of research topics. Research was seen as being primarily responsive to theoretical concerns and developments within the discipline and there was no conception that anthropological theory could be developed through a praxis outside that of traditional fieldwork[12] such as contributing practically to the welfare of those who were weak, vulnerable and easily deprived of their rights. Indeed had one been operating with an integrated consciousness that accepted that knowledge could be generated from feeling and that action in turn must follow from knowledge, the life of young women in the villages could not possibly have escaped serious attention.

The state of segregation of the feeling from the intellect and the detachment of the intellect from the will is one which is characteristic of the individual existing in the atomized state of contemporary capitalist society. Our own socially constituted being is represented in such notions as the disinterested human observer and a value-free social science. It is my view that specialised knowledge gained by the intellect,

humanitarian concern accessible through one's feeling, and
political commitment sustained by one's will must be the
joint source of research problems.

Notes

1   This chapter emerged out of discussions I had as a postgradute
     student at Manchester University in 1968 with Dr Moshe Shokheid,
     now Reader in Social Anthropology, University of Tel Aviv, and
     the late Professor Max Gluckman. I am grateful to my many
     friends who commented subsequently, especially Rohit Barot,
     Lecturer in the Department of Sociology, University of Bristol,
     and Mae McCann, Lecturer, Department of Social Anthropology,
     Queen's University of Belfast. The chapter is written primarily in
     'a spirit of faithfulness' to those young Jat women whom I knew
     and who pictured their life as a constant experience of humiliation.
     Among these it is especially for my sister-in-law, Jasminder. Rural
     Jat society indeed expressed itself through the sufferings of these
     women and in its treatment of their feelings.

2   'Researchers in the Social Sciences are faced with a unique
     methodological problem; the very conditions of their research
     constitute an important complex variable for what passes as the
     findings of their investigations. Field research . . . is a method in
     which the activities of the investigator play a crucial role in the
     data obtained' (Cicourel, 1964, p.39).

3   'He is the project . . . he is the information absorber, the informa-
     tion analyser, the information synthesizer and information inter-
     preter. . . . the critical tool in anthropological research is the
     researcher himself' (Freilich, 1970, pp.32–3).

4   'The person facing fieldwork for the first time . . . may suspect
     ethnographers of having established a conspiracy of silence on
     these matters. . . . As a result of the rules of the game which kept
     others from communicating their experience to him, he may feel
     that his own difficulties of morale and rapport . . . were unique
     and perhaps signs of weakness or incompetence. Consequently,
     these are concealed or minimized' (Berreman, 1962, p.4).

5   This confirms Vidich's reflection (1955, p.354) that 'what an
     observer will see will depend largely on his particular position in
     a network of relations.'

6   In this context one can note Dean's statement in Doby (1954,
     p.233): 'A person becomes accepted as a participant observer
     more because of the kind of person he turns out to be in the eyes
     of field contacts than because of what the research means to
     them.' See also in this connection Whyte (1965, p.300).

7   Many years later I was reminded of these feelings when I read *A*

Village in Anatolia (Makal, 1954). The author describes how a husband takes his wife to the doctor and thinks that since he has come to the town after such a long time he should also buy her some sweetmeats. He walks on ahead, but she does not follow because she has to pass a group of men. When he turns, he sees her standing with her face to the wall.

8   *Jatti* is the female for Jat, and it means here a woman belonging to the landowning section of the Sikh community.

9   Lévi-Strauss (1967, p.26) therefore does justice to the drama of the situation when he speaks of 'the servility of observation as it is practised by the anthropologist. Leaving his country and his home for long periods . . . allowing his habits, his beliefs, and his convictions to be tampered with, conniving at this, indeed, when without mental reservations or ulterior motives, he assumes the mode of life of a strange society, the anthropologist practises total observation, beyond which there is nothing except — and there is a risk — the complete absorption of the observer by the object of his observations.'

10   The experience was a very obvious instance of the beneficial consequence of stress. For a discussion of stress in a fieldwork situation see Winthrob's article in Henry and Saberwal (eds), *Stress and Response in Fieldwork* (1969).

11   It is therefore interesting to read that John Honigman (1957) has recorded in a footnote at the close of an article on women in Pakistan that 'The reader will gather from this paper that a male anthropologist had little opportunity to directly study women's roles'.

12   In paediatrics, for example, the theoretical assessment of doctor-value has taken into practical consideration community needs. Medical priorities which traditionally gave primacy to research now regard capability of service as of equal importance, (see Morley, 1973).

References

Berreman, G.D. (1962), *Behind Many Masks*, Society for Applied Anthropology, Monograph No. 4, Cornell University Press, Ithaca, New York.

Beteille, A. and Madan, T.N. (eds) (1976), *Encounter and Experience*, Vikas, New Delhi.

Cicourel, A.V. (1964), *Method and Measurement in Sociology*, Free Press, New York.

Dean, J.P. (1954), 'Participant Observation and Interviewing' in John T. Doby (ed.), *Introduction to Social Research*, Harrisburg, Pa., The Stackpole Company.

Evans-Pritchard, E.E. (1964), *Social Anthropology*, Cohen & West, London.

Fernea, E. and Bezirgan, B.Q. (eds) (1976), *Middle Eastern Muslim Women Speak*, University of Texas Press, Austin.

Freilich, M. (1970), *Marginal Natives. Anthropologists at Work*, Harper & Row, New York.

Henry, F. and Saberwal, S. (eds) (1969), *Stress and Response in Fieldwork*, Holt, Rinehart & Winston, New York.

Honigmann, J.J. (1957), 'Woman in West Pakistan' in Maron (ed.), *Pakistan Society and Culture*, Human Relations Area Files, Yale University Press, New Haven, pp.154-76.

Jacobson, Doranne (1976), 'The Veil of Virtue: Purdah and the Muslim Family in the Bhopal Region of Central India', I. Ahmad (ed.), *Family and Kinship among Muslims in India*, Manohar Book Service, Delhi, pp.169-215.

Lévi-Strauss, C. (1967), *The Scope of Anthropology*, Jonathan Cape, London.

Makal, M. (1954), *A Village in Anatolia*, Valentine, Mitchell, London.

Morley, D. (1973), *Paediatric Priorities in the Developing World*, Butterworth, London.

Papanek, H. (1964), 'The Woman Fieldworker in a Purdah Society', *Human Organisation*, vol. 23 pp.160-3.

Papanek, H. (1973), 'Purdah: Separate Worlds and Symbolic Shelter', *Comparative Studies in Society and History*, vol. 15, pp.289-325.

Pettigrew, J.J.M. (1971), *The Emigration of Sikh Jats from the Punjab to England*, Report for the Social Science Research Council, London.

Pettigrew, J.J.M. (1975), *Robber Noblemen*, Routledge & Kegan Paul, London.

Sturtevant, W.C. (1967), 'Urgent Anthropology', Report on the Smithsonian-Wenner Gren Conference, *Current Anthropology*, vol. 8, no. 4, pp.255-9.

Vidich, A.J. (1955), 'Participant Observation and the Collection and Interpretation of Data', *American Journal of Sociology*, no. 60, pp.354-60.

Whyte, W.F. (1965), *Street Corner Society*, University of Chicago Press, Appendix, pp.279-356.

4

Men, masculinity and the process of sociological enquiry

David Morgan

In this chapter, David Morgan re-examines some of his own work in the light of the feminist critique, and in doing so asks to what extent the dominant rationality in sociology is a 'male rationality'. In approaching this question, he suggests that a tentative distinction may be made between, first, formal/ academic/scholarly/scientific rationality concerning matters such as 'reliability', 'validity', 'falsifiability', 'verifiability', 'bias', 'objectivity', in other words the various claims and counter-claims by which sociological work is evaluated; and second, the substantive culture of academic, or more specifi- cally sociological rationality, i.e. the symbols, rituals and regular routinised practices which indicate ways of doing rationality. Morgan suggests that, in principle, the claims of formal academic rationality are not gender-bound, with the possible and important exception of the question of the use of personal experience in sociological accounts, but that at the level of culture, the model of rationality becomes confounded with the dominant male culture of the university environment.

Morgan argues that considerations of gender are important to all sociological research from the point of view of scholar- ship as well as from an ethical or a political point of view, but suggests that the structure of existing academic institutions militates against change.

83

I think he be transformed into a beast;
For I can nowhere find him like a man.
(*As You Like It*)

This chapter came about as the result of two events. In the first place, and most immediately, Helen Roberts persuaded me to contribute to a session on 'non-sexist methodology' at a conference on methodology organised by the British Sociological Association and Social Science Research Council in January 1979.[1] Since the term 'non-sexist methodology' presents all kinds of conceptual and methodological difficulties (some of which I indicate later) I shall not make it the central theme of this particular chapter which is more to do with the way in which notions of 'men' and 'masculinity' pervade sociological enquiry and the way in which these might be related to the conditions of production of academic work. A second, and possibly deeper influence, one which certainly influenced my decision to agree to participate in the 'non-sexist methodology' session, was my experiences as a tutor at the BSA Summer School on 'Feminism and Sociological Research' in the Summer of 1978. To use Frankenberg's distinction,[2] this was closer to 'knowing' than to 'knowing about'. I had 'known about' feminism before participating in the Summer School and I had some thoughts about its relationship to sociological theorising. But to participate in a conference where the two men tutors[3] and the three or four men students were very much outnumbered by a largely feminist population was a much more profound form of 'knowing'. This was not, let me stress, the result of any overt hostility. On the contrary, I reflected that, had the gender-ratio been reversed I should have been either propositioned or patronised and, in any event, largely excluded. Rather, what happened was that, at each point, my normally-taken-for-granted gender came up for critical self-examination and reflection. For a while the experience which is, I suspect, the lot of most women academics for most of the time was in some small way my experience.

By way of approaching this topic consider the following two extracts taken from one of the most celebrated methodological appendices in the history of empirical sociology (Whyte, 1943, pp.302, 299):

Whenever a girl or a group of girls would walk down the street, the fellows on the corner would make mental notes and later would discuss their evaluations of the females. These evaluations would run largely in terms of shape, and here I was glad to argue that Mary had a better 'build' than Anna or vice versa.

As I went along, I found that life in Cornerville was not nearly so interesting and pleasant for the girls as it was for the men. A young man had complete freedom to wander and hang around. The girls could not hang on street corners.

These are clearly not unambiguously 'sexist' passages. Certainly Whyte appears to have been 'glad' to compare the shapes of Mary and Anna and this may suggest a zeal beyond the demands of rapport. Certainly he uses the term 'girl' without indicating whether it is a native term or whether the implicit bracketing of woman/child is his own work. And yet the passages could be treated as much as a demonstration of the part that sexism plays in a particular social setting including a recognition of the constraints that it places on women's freedom of movement, as a manifestation of implicit sexism. And yet again the book, which treats largely of the affairs of men and masculinity is called *Street Corner Society*. Perhaps the infrequency with which women appear in the book is a reflection of Whyte's own difficulties as a male investigator or of the actual situation which obtained in Cornerville or, most likely, both of these in interaction. The point is not whether Whyte and his book may be correctly labelled as 'sexist' but to consider the process whereby considerations of gender failed to occupy a central place in the book and in most subsequent discussions of it.

It is a measure of the worth of Whyte's book that we may possibly recover some of the answers to questions about gender from the text even if they did not form the central theme of the research. Clearly most sociological texts have some degree of ambiguity in this respect and it was partly for this reason that I decided to abandon, as a central concern, the question of 'sexist' versus 'non-sexist' methodology. There were two further difficulties. In the first place, the term 'non-sexist methodology' implied that there was some absolute standard of objectivity by which sociological research could be evaluated. Few sociologists, I suspect, would accept this assumption in other areas and there seemed to be little point in introducing it in a discussion of sexism and sociological research. The term 'less-sexist methodology' might possibly recommend itself as a substitute but I do not intend to use it at all systematically in this chapter. In the second place, there was the problem of this distinction between 'feminist' and 'non-sexist' methodology.[4] Clearly, the distinction can and should be made and that the former term, since it is more positive and more precise, is to be preferred. If, however, this term is to be preserved, we are faced with the further problem as to whether men could ever be considered as undertaking feminist research.

In the light of these difficulties I consider my aim in this chapter to be a relatively modest one. I am taking for granted the feminist critique of everyday sociological practice — whether in research or teaching, theorising or empirical research — and am seeking to ask, in the light of this critique, what are the implications for male researchers, for men in sociology? I hope to illustrate some of these themes from examples taken from my own work and I attempt to situate this discussion in an examination of the normal conditions of academic sociological enquiry.[5]

I should stress at the beginning that I am not arguing for or against the adoption of particular techniques or modes of sociological enquiry; rather I am arguing for a critical examination of the social context of sociological research, the assumptions that arise out of this context and the way in which these assumptions (by their silences and omissions as much as by their more obvious statements) shape the more detailed processes of enquiry. In other words, I am assuming that there is nothing inherently sexist in the use of social surveys or path analysis or, indeed, in positivism.[6] Thus, while there may well be something sexist in the use of the actual terms 'hard' and 'soft' data we cannot assume that the use of 'softer' methods is in some way less sexist than the use of techniques which might be labelled 'hard'.[7] Qualitative methodology and ethnography after all has its own brand of *machismo* with its image of the male sociologist bringing back news from the fringes of society, the lower depths, the mean streets, areas traditionally 'off limits' to women investigators. What I am suggesting we need to do is to consider, to adapt a term from Eagleton,[8] the 'sociological mode of production' rather than particular methods of data collection.

It is worth stressing also that this concern about sexism in sociological enquiry is a concern about scholarship. This is not to privilege scholarship over or against the ethical or political concerns that gave rise to the debate about sexism. Indeed the way in which distinctions such as that between the scholarly and the political are made and sustained is itself a proper matter for scholarly investigation. What I am arguing, more prosaically, is that this is not just a matter of concern for those who happen to be interested in feminism or 'women's studies' but something that affects everyone engaged in sociological work. Sexist domain assumptions, in whatever specialised field of enquiry, do have consequences for the outcome of investigations and in many cases the final outcome would have been very different had the investigator taken account of questions of gender. The exacting demands of Schutz may serve as some kind of signpost for our investigations (1972, p.222):

> In scientific judgment no presupposition or any pregiven element can be accepted as simply 'at hand' without need of any further explanation. On the contrary, when I act as a scientist, I subject to a detailed step-by-step analysis everything taken from the world of everyday life: my own judgments, the judgments of others which I have previously accepted without criticism, indeed everything that I have previously taken as a matter of belief or have even thought in a confused fashion.

I hope to illustrate these assumptions as well as progress towards some tentative conclusions by examining some examples taken from my own work. In this I am following the example set by Frankenberg (Frankenberg, 1976) and the relatively simple precept that 'sexism begins at home' rather than making any particular claims about my own work as 'sexist', 'less-sexist' or 'non-sexist'.

Anglican bishops

My master's thesis was on the social and educational backgrounds of Anglican bishops from 1860 to 1960 (Morgan 1963; 1969b). In this I noted the striking although not unexpected homogeneity in terms of family background and education and the ways in which these patterns had changed or remained relatively stable over my hundred-year period. Following 'normal' sociological practice, family background was evaluated largely in terms of the status of the father. I did not, of course, note the fact of homogeneity in terms of gender. In common with most other investigations of elites in contemporary society I took this for granted as a fact so obvious that it was not worthy of comment. Similarly women appear chiefly, and briefly, as 'celebrities' in Mills's *The Power Elite* and the theme of gender is touched upon in only one paper (Kelsall's re-examination of higher civil servants) in two collections dealing with elites and power in British society.[9]

In the case of bishops, to repeat, it might appear to be labouring the obvious even to mention their homogeneity in terms of gender; to which one can only reply that the obvious deserves at least as much attention from the sociologist as the extraordinary. It is also more difficult to recognise. Furthermore, even to raise this as an issue would be also to raise a host of other interesting issues focusing on the inter-relationships between religion, gender and sexuality. Finally, if it be a reasonable assumption that a bishop's class and status backgrounds in some way shape his views on ethical or political matters it is at least as reasonable to suppose that the massive maleness of the episcopacy and the clergy generally should have an influence equal to that of economic and social status. It was often reported, for example, that Bishop X or Archbishop Y did not 'suffer fools gladly' and it would be interesting to speculate how far this was a 'masculine' trait in episcopal robes. Women, it may be hypothesised, are often expected to suffer fools gladly or at least quietly.

Somewhat more to my credit I did note that 88 per cent of the diocesan bishops during this hundred-year period were married. It did not appear to be the case that, generally speaking, a 'good' marriage directly helped preferment; in my somewhat humourless way I noted that 'bishops tend to marry in a horizontal social direction'. However the fact of marriage was clearly important to the social position of bishops just as it was, and is, to the incumbents of many other elite positions. In a recent study, Kanter shows how the proportion of managers married (and married to wives who do not hold a full-time paid job) rises with income and status (Kanter, 1977, p.28). Furthermore, marriage could be seen as reflecting a continuation of a cumulative process of immersion and involvement in a wider elite network, one which may sometimes have had consequences for preferment but almost certainly had consequences for general social and political orientations.

I did, further, have a couple of pages on the role and status of bishops' wives. This rather brief consideration did in fact slightly over-represent the treatment of the topic in the available literature at the time. I noted the frequent use of the term 'helpmeet' in episcopal biographies and autobiographies and recorded the following two quotations: 'Of course at a certain age, when you have a house and so on, you get a wife as part of the furniture and find that you have a very comfortable institution' (Creighton, 1913, p.33); 'No one, of course, could fail to observe how helpful Mrs. Wordsworth was to her husband in his new sphere; but she was so quiet and unassuming that her personality seemed to be almost merged in his' (Overton and Wordsworth, 1888, chapter 8). Yet in spite of one or two passing suggestions the role of marriage in the performance of the episcopal role remained a relatively unexplored theme in my thesis as in many other elite studies of the time. Similarly the role of marriage and kinship in elite formation, maintenance, reproduction and ideology and the way in which kinship networks change as the nature of elites change is still, with the exception of studies such as that of Lupton and Wilson, an under-explored theme (Lupton and Wilson, 1959).

A factory study

My doctoral thesis was based upon a participant observation study of a northern factory (Morgan 1969a; 1972, 1975; Emmett and Morgan, 1979). It arose out of a team project (financed by the then Department of Scientific and Industrial Research) and the other team members were Isabel Emmett, who studied managers within the same factory, and Michael Walker, who worked in a machine shop. Largely by chance I found myself working in an electrical components assembly department, consisting almost entirely of women. Men were found to be in charge of things, as managers, foremen or charge-hands or in some scientific staff capacity or, in one case, as an odd job man. The labour force of assemblers, painters, packers, testers and lower level supervisors were women.

If women were largely absent from the study of bishops they could scarcely be ignored in a factory of this kind and, indeed, the question of gender became a central concern of my thesis. Or rather, the question of women became a central concern, the way in which feminine or domestic identities became realised or significant on the shop floor; the question of men or masculine identities in the workplace was much less systematically explored, although not ignored completely. I think that I, at least initially, too readily assumed that the fact that these workers were women was a significant independent variable and that it was possible to see, or to assume, the simple carrying over of domestic identities on to the shop floor. However, as a team we were moving towards a more interactionist perspective. Characteristics such as age and gender were not seen as characteristics that automatically had an effect simply by virtue of the fact of their presence; we tended to see these as latent characteristics which were realised or muted in particular contexts, which were shaped in particular directions and combinations by these contexts and which were sometimes consequential and at other times of little consequence. In short, age and gender were not independent variables as appears to be the assumption in many statistical tables where data are broken down by age and sex. It is tempting to argue that we saw age and gender as dependent variables but the very use of these terms would be out of keeping with the spirit of an interactionist approach. Gender became important in a particular way, when, for example, an unmarried, personable male supervisor was attempting to coax work out of unmarried, personable female employees; gender becomes significant in different ways when that same supervisor was dealing with an older, married female employee.

It is worth noting the way in which participant observation contributed to this way of seeing gender as something shaped and patterned in interactional contexts rather than as something unchanging that is brought to every encounter. As a man, I was very conscious of my ambiguous position in the department. My gender placed me —in that context —in the same position as the foreman and managers. The occupational role that I had assumed while carrying out the research, on the other hand placed me in the same position as the female employees. My class — reflected chiefly in my accent and my connections with the university — served to distance me from both categories. Age and marital status were yet further additional factors; some women at least were able to neutralise some of the ambiguities in my status in the department by adopting a quasi-maternal role, expressing concern about how I managed on my own and, in one case, offering to wash my shirts for me. This was not simply a case of a man working among women; it was a case of a man with various other characteristics working in a particular department — with a particular labour force composition. In a different department — say the one that encountered another male colleague who worked on the project for a short while and was placed in a section employing a high proportion of young unmarried women — different latent characteristics would have come to the fore. The point I want to stress here is that gender differences in fieldwork are not simply a source of difficulties such as exclusion from important central rituals or, in my case, exclusion from all-important interactions in the toilets, but are also a source of knowledge about the particular field. The 'participant observer', in short, has a gender identity.

Bloomsbury

I am currently attempting a study of Bloomsbury, using the abundant and ever-growing published literature to explore

various themes in my overlapping interests in the sociology of
the family and the sociology of culture. One theme that I have
been exploring is that of 'friendship', its meaning and significance, its relationship to the processes of cultural production,
and the way in which, in this particular grouping, a certain
ideology of friendship could have been said to have been ela-
borated. One of the aspects of this ideology appears to have
been a belief in the possibility of friendship between men and
women, friendship that was not necessarily confounded by
sexual attractions or jealousies. My early source for this theme
was the set of volumes of reminiscences by Leonard Woolf
and subsequent writings and commentaries (by authors such
as Michael Holroyd, writing on Strachey) seemed to confirm
this picture. It is only recently, in reading the first volume of
letters by Virginia Woolf, that I have realised that this may
have been a male perspective on friendship relationships
(Nicolson (ed.), 1975). Here she expresses a degree of exclusion from and perhaps even some distaste for the conversations of the Cambridge Apostles who gathered in Bloomsbury.
Her letters to women show a much greater freedom and spontaneity than, for the most part, her letters to men. This
impression is confirmed in Showalter's critical assessment of
the Bloomsbury group and her argument that, in the accounts
of the circumstances surrounding Virginia Woolf's 'break-
downs' and ultimate suicide, there is the danger that Leonard's
version might prevail over that of Virginia (Showalter, 1978,
p.279). This work is still in progress but it would appear that
Jessie Bernard's question — 'whose marriage?' (Bernard, 1973)
— has relevance here and that we should also ask the equally
pertinent question, 'whose friendship?'

There is one not insignificant footnote — a reminder to
myself, as it were — to this brief account of my work on
Bloomsbury. Just as 'men who manage', often manage with
the aid of a largely unheralded grouping of women in the role
of secretaries (a point only recently given the recognition it
deserves by Kanter (Kanter, 1977, pp.69–103)) so too these
open and formally egalitarian relationships between friends
were supported by a hidden stage crew of servants, again largely female (Davidoff, 1974).

The Protestant Ethic and the Spirit of Capitalism

Finally I turn, with what might seem to be almost indecent abruptness, from a consideration of my own work to a very brief consideration of one of the classical texts in sociology: Weber's *Protestant Ethic and the Spirit of Capitalism*. It cannot have escaped many people's attention, at least in recent years, that women are very much hidden from this particular history; the lead parts — Franklin, Luther, Calvin, Baxter and Wesley — are all played by men and women only appear on the stage fleetingly in the guise of German factory workers with rather traditional orientations to work. Yet here, as elsewhere, these silences and omissions have their own eloquence. We are told how capitalist rationality required the separation of the workplace and household, a commonplace that has formed the background (perhaps too readily) for the examination of domestic labour under capitalism. Further, an important sub-theme in this text is the re-definition of sexuality and the way in which this became defined as a force most at odds with bourgeois rationality. If sexuality became identified with the irrational it is easy to see how it was possible for both to become identified with women, largely excluded from the main public arena of capitalist enterprise.

But most of all, perhaps, it is possible to see Weber's *Protestant Ethic* as a study of masculinity, not a universal, biologically fixed notion of masculinity but one that was intimately bound up with the developing social formation of capitalism. The main character traits of the ideal-typical puritan — self-control, discipline, rationality, methodicalness — are traits which would probably be defined as 'masculine' by many people, including not a few social psychologists, in contemporary society. Contemporary feminist theory has been much concerned with the interplay of patriarchy and capitalism and it is likely that a re-examination of Weber's study could provide some fascinating insights into this complex area (Hamilton, 1978, chapter 3; Hoch, 1979, chapter 9). In this study, as in many other studies, men were there all the time but we did not see them because we imagined that we were looking at mankind.

This kind of re-analysis could, of course, be continued at much greater length and in much greater depth. I hope that I have provided enough to serve as illustrative material for a variety of interlinking general themes.

1   In the first place, I hope that I have demonstrated the need for taking gender seriously. If it is possible to talk of a non-sexist or less-sexist methodology, this must be the first requirement. Furthermore, 'taking gender seriously' is not simply a recognition of the justice of the feminist charges aginst normal sociological practice, perhaps a grudging or a mechanical recognition, but an exploration that can raise new issues and point the way to new solutions. It is, in short, a scholarly requirement, let alone anything else.

Yet it can also be seen that 'taking account of gender' is by no means a simple operation, the addition of one more category of analysis. It means taking account, reflexively, of the gender of the researcher, as well as of the researched, and of the two in interaction. It involves, too, a critical examination of the notions of gender differentiation as they enter into sociological analysis, an examination of the routine assumptions that may lie behind the breaking down of numerical data 'by sex' (Mathieu, 1977; Oakley and Oakley, 1979). It involves devising modes of sociological or historical enquiry which may begin to capture the lives of those who are often 'hidden from history' — in the examples used here, the servants and the wives.

2   It may be noted that where gender is 'taken into account' it is usually in relation to women; I only started to consider gender to any real extent when I found myself in a factory department consisting largely of women. The same of course is true of whites and gentiles as opposed to blacks and Jews. We know more about wives and mothers than about husbands and fathers; if the former are obscured from our vision by being too far in the background, the latter are obscured from our vision by being, like Weber's Prostestants, too much in the foreground. When I started to think about my field-data I turned to the existing literature, even then quite extensive, dealing with 'women at work', work which treated this as a problem to be explained or justified. Consequently, I

attempted to seek out ways in which feminine or domestic identities became manifest in the workplace. My analysis of masculinity was much more muted, although not entirely absent. Following the lead provided by Willis in his discussion of sexism among male adolescents and the way in which this sexism is part of the process of 'learning to labour' or the process whereby working-class kids get working-class jobs, it should be possible to re-examine some classic workshop ethnographies (Willis, 1978). A good candidate for such re-analysis might be Donald Roy's study of horseplay on the shopfloor, 'Banana Time', and not simply for the more obvious phallic connotations (Roy, 1960). Most workshop ethnographies — and other studies of occupations — are normally about men anyway and the re-examination of these studies in the light of notions of gender and masculinity should prove to be an illuminating, if difficult task. Thus taking gender into account is 'taking men into account' and not treating them — by ignoring the question of gender — as the normal subjects of research.

3   Moving away, a little, from the illustrative material it may be argued that 'taking gender into account' is particularly a problem for male sociologists. This is not to say that women in sociology have not, at times, been equally guilty of ignoring gender or of treating it as a one sided question of 'women in society'.[10] Women may be under internal or external pressure as 'tokens' or 'minorities'[11] to avoid gender issues or to treat them in the conventional manner. Yet, at the time of writing, women are more likely to see the connections between their own experiences as students, post-graduates, researchers and staff members in academic and research institutions on the one hand and the work arising out of the women's movement on the other. The BSA Women's Caucus is, it would appear from the outside, one such point of articulation between the two. Men, on the other hand, have to work against the grain — their grain — in order to free their work from sexism, to take gender into account. The male researcher needs, as it were, a small voice at his shoulder reminding him at each point that he is a man. As the examples from my own work demonstrate — and I doubt whether they are atypical in this respect at least — the massive weight of the taken-for-granted

(probably the most pervasive domain assumption) conspires with the researcher's own gender to render silent what should be spoken.

4   When we begin to account for the partial and often inadequate treatment of gender in sociological research, it is clearly not enought to blame particular techniques of data collection, particularly those which are conventionally identified with 'positivism'. Nor is it enough to say — as it may be said in some of the less illuminating exchanges of the sex-war at the inter-personal level — 'because you are a man'. We need, rather, to look at the context of sociological work, at the sociological mode of production. Here, I begin to consider the assumptions behind normal sociological enquiry, the processes by which genuine or authentic sociological work comes to be recognised as such and the role that these processes play in the elaboration and financing of research projects. Awareness of the political context of sociology — among other disciplines — is not, of course, a novelty. There may be some dispute, to put the matter gently, as to the extent to which and the way in which universities may be described as 'ideological state apparatuses' or as 'servicing capitalism'. Yet the sociologies of knowledge and science, whether or not informed by Marxism, have rendered the model of the university as an arena for the disinterested pursuit and dissemination of scholarship an even more improbable model of reality.One only has to consider the complex ways in which the divorce between mental and manual labour both shapes and is shaped by the processes of scholarly enquiry within universities and other institutions.

Part of this political context of sociological enquiry must continue to be the male dominance of the universities. Table 4.1, taken from an AUT *Bulletin*, presents the general picture. Dominance is not merely a numerical matter; one woman appears on the list of names of current members of Council at Manchester University and only a handful of women's names appear on the list of 250 plus who are members of Senate.[12] Women, in Kanter's terms, are still 'tokens' or 'minorities' in most university departments. I am not concerned here to present these facts in any more detail or to elaborate on the complex patterns of causes that have led to this continuing

Table 4.1 *Women in British universities*

Grade	Men	Women	Total	% of women
Professors	4,121	84	4,205	2.0
Readers, Senior Lecturers	7,647	499	8,146	6.1
Lecturers, Assistant Lecturers	21,288	3,260	24,548	13.3
Others (research staff, etc. majority paid beneath Lecturer minimum)	1,585	642	2,227	28.8
Totals	34,641	4,485	39,126	11.5

% of men above Lecturer grade out of total men employed	34%
% of women above Lecturer grade out of total women employed	13%

Source: AUT *Bulletin*, June 1978, p.14.

imbalance. I am here more concerned with suggesting what may be the consequences of such an imbalance. I am arguing, therefore, that it is not just a statistical index of discrimination but a structural feature that affects the whole business of scholarship and teaching. The question I am asking is one of how far the academic discourse is in fact a male discourse, sheltering behind such labels as 'rationality', 'scientific' or 'scholarly'?

This is not a new question. A reviewer, writing about Adrienne Rich's *Of Woman Born*, puts the issue in its starkest form (Galloway, December 1978; her emphasis):

> Feminists have recognised for some time that one of the primary characteristics of the man-made culture is the insistence that the 'personal' be separated from the 'political' in all forms of social analysis: 'motherhood' can only be studied 'objectively' (i.e. as a *fact* which exists *independently* of personal experience) as an 'institution'. The male demand for 'objectivity' is, of course, no more than an arrogant claim for the exlusive legitimacy of their own subjective awareness (i.e. motherhood is seen in the context of *their* needs).

This is clearly a much wider question than the gender imbalance within universities; it is to do with the 'maleness' of
culture and language. Even within the more limited scope of
this paper, to argue for the complete or near-complete
relativisation of sociological knowledge on gender lines, to
make claims for a feminist way of knowing or seeing against
a dominant masculine way of seeing, is to open up a complex
series of questions in the sociology of knowledge which reflect
but also cut across similar problems raised by the Marxist
critique of bourgeois social science.[13] These would include
the nature and boundaries of the social entity (class, biological
sex or cultural gender) within which the hegemonic culture
and knowledge is located, the way in which this culture is accepted or internalised by those outside and subordinate to
those entities, the way in which oppositional versions of reality
are generated and sustained and the extent to which it is possible to adjudicate between alternative versions of reality.

There is not the space nor do I feel competent to discuss
the complex philosophical ramifications of this particular
version of the relativism debate. It is enough at this stage
merely to remind ourselves that these complexities exist.
However, one tentative distinction, with some bearing on
the argument of this paper, may be attempted. On the one
hand we may posit a cluster of terms to indicate a pattern we
may call 'sociological rationality', itself a sub-set of academic
or scholarly rationality. Among these terms we may note
'reliability', 'validity', 'falsifiability', 'verifiability', 'internal
consistency' and so on. These, and similar terms, are the staple
diet of methodology textbooks and refer to the criteria by
which sociological practices may be evaluated, by which,
indeed, pieces of work may be said to 'count' as sociology.
While there may well be competing claims made on behalf of
or against particular sociological practices within this framework of sociological rationality, the claims and counter-claims
are, in principal, largely non-gender-specific. This is not to say
that this whole framework may not, in some wider sense, be
seen as culture bound and that this culture will include, as
one of its major themes, patriarchy. Yet, within this somewhat
narrower, more specific framework it can be argued that there
are questions which one would wish to ask of, say, Oakley's

Sociology of Housework which are of the same order as the questions we would wish to ask of Young and Willmott's *The Symmetrical Family* or the Pahls' *Managers and their Wives.* These are the more or less standard questions about the relationships between the methods adopted, the data collected and presented and the conclusions drawn and the underlying assumptions, implicit or explicit, that shape all of these.

I am aware that this characterisation of sociological rationality is a little vague, and this is probably necessarily so. In a sense the nature of this rationality only emerges through the detailed examination of actual sociological practice, the reports of findings, the conferences, the seminar papers and the book reviews. What I have in mind is probably best described by E.P. Thompson in his discussion of 'historical logic':[14]

> By 'historical logic' I mean a logical method of enquiry appropriate to historical materials, designed as far as possible to test hypotheses as to structure, causation, etc., and to eliminate self-confirming procedures ('instances', 'illustrations'). The disciplined historical discourse of the proof consists in a dialogue between concept and evidence, a dialogue conducted by successive hypotheses, on the one hand, and empirical research on the other. . . . To name this logic is not, of course, to claim that it is always evidenced in every historian's practice, or in any historian's practice all of the time . . . . But it is to say that this logic does not disclose itself involuntarily; that the discipline requires arduous preparation; and that three thousand years of practice have taught us something. And it is to say that it is this logic which constitutes the discipline's ultimate court of appeal: *not*, please note, 'the evidence' by itself, but the evidence interrogated thus.

It is perhaps chastening to substitute the term 'sociological logic' (or 'sociological rationality') for Thompson's 'historical logic'; to remind ourselves that sociological work is always flawed and partial and certainly ardous.

There is one possible exception to this characterisation of sociological rationality as being in principle non-gender-specific and that is in the area of personal experience. On the whole, sociologists have been at pains to distance their undertakings from personal experience, perhaps bracketing it with 'common sense' and other sources of contamination. In so doing, sociologists may often claim, with some justice, to be performing a liberating function. An undergraduate who makes claims about the openness of the British class system on the grounds that she/he as a working-class kid managed to get to university will be directed to Westergaard and Resler. The feminist movement, on the other hand, has introduced a new emphasis in sociological enquiry reflecting the slogan 'the personal is the political' and incorporating autobiographical and literary material into sociological accounts. My belief is that these perspectives, the feminist emphasis on 'the personal' and my characterisation of sociological rationality are not necessarily irreconcilable and that there is a lot of work to be done in exploring the relationships between various forms of social knowledge such as personal experience, fictional representations and sociological enquiry. This work is or should be part of sociological rationality. A recent valuable contribution to this part of the debate is provided by Stanley and Wise in their examination of the complex relationship between feminist consciousness and experience of sexism in their personal encounter with obscene telephone calls (Stanley and Wise, 1979).

Yet this typification of sociological rationality is not the whole story. At the same time, and inextricably intermingled with the business of sociological evaluation, is a culture of sociological (or academic) rationality, a set of symbols, rituals and regular routinised practices which indicate ways of being rational or perhaps ways of doing rationality. In addition this culture will influence the process by which research topics and modes of investigation are negotiated. It is at this point that the rational merges with the masculine, that the practice of sociological (or any other, for that matter) enquiry blends with the dominant male culture of the university environment. Here I am re-emphasising the point that we are not dealing with a simple statistical imbalance but that the dominance of

men in academic settings creates something which we call a
'male culture' although it is usually inarticulated as such and
rarely recognised. It is of course one of the contributions of
the feminist movement and of the personal experiences of
women in academic settings that we are now able, if
imperfectly, to recognise some features of this male culture.
In case, in what is to follow, I may appear to be adopting an
'holier than thou' attitude towards my male colleagues let
me say that I am describing practices and attitudes which I
recognise within myself and in which I have participated.

It is at this point, then, I would like to introduce the notion
of 'academic *machismo*'. The arenas of the practice of
academic rationality – the seminars, the conferences, the
exchanges in scholarly journals – are also arenas for the competitive display of masculine skills (within, to be sure, a capitalist culture), a display which may be the more deadly since
it is carried on in the partial realisation of the popular stereo-
type of the academic as someone who could not 'make it' (in
all senses) in the real world, as someone essentially desiccated
and sexless.[15] Consider the phrases which are often used to
describe academic exchanges – 'wiped the floor with him',
'tore him into little pieces' and so on – phrases more redolent
of gladiatorial combat than scholarly debate.[16] The symbolic
leaders or academic folk heroes are sharp, quick on the draw,
masters of the deadly put-down, and form the subject of
admiring gossip and recollection in the staff clubs and senior
common-rooms for some months after the original exchange.
Ellmann, although not writing primarily about academics, is
apt here (1968, p.23):

> the male mind . . . is assumed to function primarily like
> a penis. Its fundamental character is seen to be aggression,
> and this quality is held essential to the highest or best
> working of the intellect. Jobs must be tackled, objec-
> tions overruled, problems attacked, difficulties overcome
> and offensives must always be seized.

I suspect that most readers could supply examples of this
academic *machismo* in action (Silverstein, 1975). Atkinson's
description of a first publication serving 'a ritual integrative

function similar to being blooded during a fox hunt' might serve (Atkinson, 1977, p.41) but I prefer the following description of seminars at Manchester during the time of W.J.M. Mackenzie: 'They were, indeed, a formidable group of scholars, of powerful mind, strong personality and occasionally sharp tongue, who could stimulate but sometimes intimidate. More than one visiting academic who addressed a Manchester seminar found it a traumatic experience' (Birch and Spann, 1974, p.3). It is perhaps not surprising that we read later that Mackenzie built his department 'by appointing the most talented young *men* he could find, with a wide variety of backgrounds and interests, in the hope that they would strike sparks off one another and create an atmosphere of intellectual excitement' (*ibid.*, p.7, my emphasis). Perhaps another version of this academic *machismo* is the tight-lipped and largely humourless wit displayed at Senate meetings and other ritual occasions by what E.P. Thompson described as 'fully grown specimens of the species *Academicus Superciliosus* '(Thompson, 1970, p.153).

It should not be thought that the introduction of women into universities necessarily alters this masculine culture. Indeed, as Kanter suggests, the introduction of women as 'tokens' or 'minorities' into large organisations has effects on both the minorities and the majorities (Kanter, 1977, pp.206–42). The women either find themselves adopting roles defined by the majority — 'mother', 'seductress', 'pet' or 'iron maiden' — or accept the rules of conduct prescribed by the dominant culture. The men perhaps define their boundaries even more sharply as a result of the presence of minorities. Kanter is describing business organisations in the USA; a similar analysis of academic institutions would be valuable.

Partially supporting and partially counterbalancing the potentially centrifugal tendencies of academic *machismo* are the more centripetal forces of male *homosociability*. This term has been developed to capture the more subtle processes of sex discrimination and exclusion that may persist under conditions of formal equality (Lipman-Blumen, 1976, p.16):

we shall define 'homosocial' as the seeking, enjoyment, and/or preference for the company of the same sex. . . .

Men can and commonly do seek satisfaction for most of their needs from other men. They can derive satisfaction for their intellectual, physical, political, economic, occupational, social, power, and status needs — and in some circumstances their sexual needs — from other men. The dominance order among men is based upon control of resources, including land, money, education, occupations, political connections, and family ties.

Male homosociability can be seen as a mechanism of social and cultural reproduction. It is based upon a collective control of resources and serves, among other things, to exclude newcomers and outsiders from gaining access to these resources. It is clear that these mechanisms need not be fully recognised or deliberate and that they can operate through the subtle closures and exclusions in everyday conversation and socialising as well as through a 'men only' sign on the door.

In academic circles, this male sociability is reflected in the easy culture of the faculty club, the staff bar or the local pub and in conversations about sport, cars or hi-fi equipment. At one level this is simply a reflection of the fact that here, and in other occupational contexts, men tend to feel more at ease in each other's company and to display degrees of inauthenticity and unease in the company of women (especially where these women are in a minority), an unease that tends to maintain social distance and male dominance of academic institutions. Thus it is still readily assumed that a seminar 'might continue in the pub' or that a departmental matter might be 'discussed over a pint' without full recognition of the fact that, to many women, pubs are still seen as male institutions, places to which they may be taken by their escorts rather than places which are authentically 'theirs'. Married women academics may well also feel the competing claims of home and family at opening time more sharply than their male collegues just as they may feel these cross-pressures at the time of conferences organised during school holidays.[17]

It should not be assumed that these patterns of sociability

simply serve expressive or emotional supportive functions.
Just as Fleet Street male journalists exchange much valuable
gossip, tips, tricks of the trade and so on in the course
of their social drinking so too do male academics gain access
to valuable career resources in the course of their informal
meetings over a pint.[18] It would be tedious and, at this
stage, impressionistic to list all these resources but it should
not be imagined that it is exhausted simply by referring
to information about jobs and publication outlets. We
must also refer to simple everyday information: who is in
charge of which committee, who to approach about leave of
absence or travelling grants, who 'knows' about overseas
students, organising conferences, audio-visual aids and
typing theses.

It should not be necessary to remind ourselves that this
account of the mode of sociological production — focusing
here on the gender dimension with its patterns of academic
machismo and male sociability — has its own hidden dimension. In the first place there are wives and lovers, in their
more-or-less traditional roles of reproducing the academic
labour force. Here, perhaps a quotation from Lukes's intellectual biography of Durkheim will have to stand in the place of
more extended analysis (Lukes, 1975, p.99):

> and of his domestic circumstances Davy has written that
> the domestic ideal that is evident in his writings (the
> family being his favourite subject of study and lecturing)
> was most clearly represented by his own home life.
> Mauss writes, similarly, that his wife 'created for him the
> respectable and quiet familiar existence which he con-
> sidered the best guarantee of morality and of life. She
> removed from him every material care and all frivolity,
> and for his sake took charge of the education of Marie
> and André Durkheim.'

In the second place, there are secretaries and typists, almost
universally female, and, at least for higher academic grades,
likely to be found performing emotional-supportive roles as
well as more material functions. This is not simply a further
manifestation of the sexual division of labour; as the Lukes

quotation suggests, whole views of the world may be influenced by these everyday conditions of academic labour.

I am aware that this analysis — if it may be called such — has already raised several difficulties. In the first place we need to consider the terms 'masculine'and 'feminine' for it may seem that I am falling a victim to these stereotypes as much as many other sociologists criticised in this and in other volumes. It should be clear, that I am not using these terms to indicate some biological or psychological imperatives or to argue for some version of the 'natural superiority of women'. I am arguing that the dominance — numerically and politically — of men in academic life has generated a culture which can be identified, in some of its manifestations, as a 'masculine' culture. I am also recognising that this label, like the original patterns of dominance, has a complex set of historical, cultural and psychological determinations. I also recognise that this 'masculine' culture combines with other features of academic culture in very complex ways.

As an illustration of this argument about the congruence between certain notions of masculinity and desired qualities in university life, it is interesting to consider the list of traits drawn up by Brim which he assigns to male (instrumental) or female (expressive) roles (Table 4.2).[19] It should be stressed that Brim does not necessarily consider these traits to be in some way 'essentially' masculine or feminine; these are merely traits which are judged to be such. On the one hand, then, we have the traits of tenacity, aggressiveness, curiosity, ambition, planfulness, responsibility, originality, competitiveness and self-confidence. (These are traits which are regarded as being congruent with instrumental roles). On the other hand, we have obedience, affectionateness, responds to sympathy and approval from adults, speedy recovery from emotional disturbance, kindness, friendliness to adults and children. As an exercise consider these following imaginary extracts from references:

> While X is clearly ambitious, some might say to the point of aggressiveness, it is clear that she/he has a lot to be ambitious about. His/her work displays constant originality combined with an analytical rigour and an exciting sense of intellectual curiosity.

Table 4.2 *Traits assignable to male (instrumental) or female (expressive) roles*

Trait name	Pertains primarily to instrumental (I) or expressive (E) role	Trait is congruent (X) or incongru- ent (−) charac- teristic of role
Tenacity	I	X
Aggressiveness	I	X
Curiosity	I	X
Ambition	I	X
Planfulness	I	X
Dawdling and procrastinating	I	−
Responsibleness	I	X
Originality	I	X
Competitiveness	I	X
Wavering in decision	I	−
Self-confidence	I	X
Anger	E	−
Quarrelsomeness	E	−
Revengefulness	E	−
Teasing	E	−
Extrapunitiveness	E	−
Insistence on rights	E	−
Exhibitionism	E	−
Un-cooperativeness with group	E	−
Affectionateness	E	X
Obedience	E	X
Upset by defeat	E	−
Responds to sympathy and approval from adults	E	X
Jealousy	E	−
Speedy recovery from emotional disturbance	E	X
Cheerfulness	E	X
Kindness	E	X
Friendliness to adults	E	X
Friendliness to children	E	X
Negativism	E	−
Tattling	E	−

Source: Orville G. Brim Jr, 'Family Structure and Sex-Role Learning by Children', reprinted in Norman W. Bell and Ezra S. Vogel, *A Modern Introduction to the Family* (rev. ed.), Free Press, 1968.

Y is a cheerful, kindly individual, always supportive, especially to new or younger members of staff. He/she has contributed a lot to the day to day working of the department, willing to accept decisions and yet displaying qualities of warmth and friendship which are always necessary in a university environment.

Who gets the job? 'A nice enough person', one can hear the committee deliberating on the seond, 'but is it *quite* what we really want?'

Of course, there are exceptions; universities are not simply or uniformly massive walls of masculinity. Departments vary as to their sex ratios; pressures on man and women vary according to their seniority; there are academic women who would rank high on Brim's instrumental/masculine characteristics; there are academic men who find much of this aspect of university culture distressing and painful: it is possible to point to all these and to many other departures from the patterns I have suggested predominate in academic life. Indeed, the interactionist perspective to which I am still, at least partially, wedded demands that we look for process of modification, negotiation, pressures for change or deflection of these pressures across the gender lines. And yet it still seems to me that universities (and possibly other institutions) have not really got round to recognising the presence of women and that while there are clearly dangers in assuming that academic rationality is completely gender-determined there are still, for the male academic, greater dangers in assuming academic rationality to be completely free of gender-specific assumptions.

In this chapter I have suggested that the now well-documented permeation of sociology by sexist background assumptions is less a product of the adoption or failure to adopt a particular methodology and much more a product of the social relations of sociological production. I have also argued that sexism is as much to do with the ways in which taken-for-granted notions of 'men' and 'masculinity' are handled in sociological enquiry, notions which are most frequently manifested in absences and silences, as it is with the way in which women are ignored or stereotyped in such work. Finally, I have attempted to argue that such considerations matter for the reason that had such assumptions and notions been confronted and explored the outcome of the enquiry under examination might have been very different or might have been the fruitful source of new lines of enquiry.

It will be clear that much of this chapter is impressionistic and polemical in tone, designed more to hint at work to be done than to present achievements accomplished. Clearly, there is still a lot of further investigation and re-analysis required. There is the task of re-assessing many strands of the sociological tradition in order to reveal the man behind the actor. In a literal sense we need to 'bring men back in'. At the same time we need to tackle the theoretical and conceptual work involved in tracing the way in which assumptions about men and masculinity enter into normal sociological enquiry. We need, further, to look more critically or reflectively at our own institutions — our universities and polytechnics — and the way in which these shape or reinforce gender assumptions.

But the work cannot stop there. For, if my assumption is correct, we need to continue to work to change the institutions within which or with the aid of which we carry out sociological enquiry. It is hardly necessary to be reminded of the work that has already come from women in this respect: without the women's movement and without work against sexism within the BSA, papers such as this would not have been written. But there are dangers in the moderate degree of success achieved by the women's movement. In some way these successes may, in the short run at least, serve to reinforce the dialectic between 'tokens' and 'dominants' outlined by Kanter: consider the arch way in which 'Ms' or 'Chairperson' may be used or that way in which remarks may be prefaced by 'I suppose I am a male chauvinist pig'. Once the course on 'Women in Society' or 'Women's Studies' has been established it is possible that it may be business as usual for the rest of us.

There may be something to be gained in men getting together to discuss these issues, not simply in order to combat some of the more overt modes of sexism but also as the beginning of ways of understanding. It may be that such meetings may begin also to exorcise that most troublesome spirit raised by Max Weber: the Protestant's sense of inner loneliness, the unseen side of the male academic culture. Yet, if it is the case that men gather together 'naturally' in any event there is always the danger that such gatherings will become yet further sources of gossip about jobs and opportunities.[20] Yet without something of this kind it is likely that we — that is male sociologists including myself — will slip back into the more familiar ways of doing things and issues of gender will once more retreat into the background.

Epilogue

Meanwhile, it is business as usual. At an SSRC Conference on graduate training in sociology (itself a largely male gathering of delegates and speakers) the air was full of references to 'chaps' and an address on current policy contained a rather confused metaphor about shaving-cream. At a follow-up conference on the teaching of methodology to graduate students one speaker claimed that he liked to 'hit' his students with Spearman's rho.

Notes

1 I am particularly grateful to Helen Roberts for her constant and kindly encouragement. Earlier versions of this chapter were presented at graduate seminars at Manchester and Bradford and also I am grateful for all the comments received on these occasions. In addition, I have received much useful advice, comment and encouragement from Sheila Allen, Colin Bell, Mike Brake, Leonore Davidoff, Margaret Hall and Peter Halfpenny.

2 Frankenburg (1979) p.14: '*Knowing* in my use implies the possibility of understanding and change. *Knowing about* does not' (his emphasis).

3 The other tutors were Jenny Shaw, Mike Brake and Diana Leonard.

4 For this distinction, see Roberts (1978). For a discussion of feminist research, see Kelly (1978).

5 One major limitation of this chapter is that it is largely confined to a discussion of sociological enquiry within universities and, indeed,

within Manchester University which may well have its own pecu-
liarities. Clearly there is scope for more comparative work.

6   This is clearly a controversial issue. For two differing views, see
      Kelly (1978) and Roberts (1978).

7   See Roberts (1978), quoting Bart, on the terminology of 'hard'
      and 'soft', *ibid.*, pp.21–2.

8   I am here adapting Eagleton's term 'literary mode of production'.
      Eagleton (1976), pp.45–48.

9   Mills (1959), chapter 4; Urry and Wakeford (1973); Stanworth
      and Giddens (1974), The paper by Kelsall — 'Recruitment to the
      Higher Civil Service — How has the Pattern Changed?' — appears
      in the last named volume, pp.170–84.

10   The recent official publication, *Marriage Matters*, ignores the dif-
      ferent experiences of marriage by men and women in spite of the
      large number of women on the committee and serving as witnesses
      (Home Office, 1979).

11   Terms used by Kanter (1977), especially pp.206–42.

12   These figures conceal one of the more bizarre features of Senate
      sittings at Manchester University. Behind the row of senior figures
      — Vice-Chancellor, Registrar, etc. — is a Victorian (?) oil painting
      of a woman, with rather improbable breasts, in a low-cut gown. A
      photograph of a contemporary sex-object would, doubtless, be
      considered tasteless.

13   A possibly old-fashioned but still extremely useful mapping of the
      issues in the sociology of knowledge is provided by Merton (1957)
      pp.456–488. See also Merton (1972) for some treatment of 'in-
      siders' and 'outsiders' in gender terms.

14   Thompson (1978) p. 231. The whole section deserves careful
      attention.

15   The emphasis on the sex lives of the central (male) protagonists in
      recent campus novels is a point worth noting in this context. I
      have in mind Malcolm Bradbury's *The History Man* and David
      Lodge's *Changing Places*.

16   See a curious paper by Holmes, 'The University Seminar and the
      Primal Horde' (Holmes, 1967). He does not consider the gender
      implications of his analysis.

17   I am grateful to Leonore Davidoff for pointing this out to me.

18   Smith (1976). I am grateful to Colin Bell for the point and the
      reference.

19   Brim, 1958, p.532. This table has already been used by Millett
      (1977) as an example of sexist assumptions in social-psychological
      research and it is worth noting that, in so far as Brim is concerned
      to show some of the social sources of gender definition within
      the family, the author may be partially exonerated from this
      charge.

20   Colin Bell drew my attention to this danger.

References

Atkinson, Maxwell (1977), 'Coroners and the Categorisation of Deaths as Suicides: Changes in Perspective as Features of the Research Process' in C. Bell and H. Newby (eds), *Doing Sociological Research*, Allen & Unwin, London, pp.31–46.

Association of University Teachers (June 1978), *Bulletin*.

Bernard, Jessie (1973), *The Future of Marriage*, Souvenir Press, London.

Birch, A.H. and Spann, R.N. (1974), 'Mackenzie at Manchester' in B. Chapman and A. Potter (eds), *W.J.M.M. Political Questions*, Manchester University Press, pp.1–23.

Brim, Orville G. Jnr (1958), 'Family Structure and Sex-Role Learning by Children', *Sociometry*, vol. XXI, pp.1–16; reprinted in Norman W. Bell and Ezra F. Vogel (eds) (1968), *A Modern Introduction to the Family* (rev. ed.), Free Press, New York, pp.526–40.

Creighton, Mandell (1913), *Life and Letters of Mandell Creighton*, Longmans Green, London.

Davidoff, Leonore (1974), 'Mastered for Life: Servant and Wife in Victorian and Edwardian England', *Journal of Social History*, vol. 7, no. 4.

Eagleton, Terry (1976), *Criticism and Ideology*, New Left Books, London.

Ellmann, Mary (1968), *Thinking about Women*, Macmillan, London.

Emmett, Isabel and Morgan, D.H.J. (1979), 'Max Gluckman and the Manchester Shop Floor Ethnographies', in Ronald Frankenberg (ed.), *Custom and Conflict in Britain*, Manchester University Press, 1981.

Frankenberg, Ronald (1976), 'In the Production of their Lives, Men (?) . . . Sex and Gender in British Community Studies' in D.L. Barker and S. Allen (eds), *Sexual Divisions and Society: Process and Change*, Tavistock, London, pp.25–51.

Frankenberg, Ronald (1979), 'Methodology: Social or Individual?', Paper read at BSA/SSRC Methodology Conference.

Galloway, Elizabeth (November/December 1978), Review of *Of Women Born* (Adrienne Rich), *WRRC Newsletter*, p.5.

Hamilton, Roberta (1978), *The Liberation of Women*, Allen & Unwin, London.

Hoch, Paul (1979), *White Hero Black Beast: Racism, Sexism and the Mask of Masculinity*, Pluto Press, London.

Holmes, Roger (1967), 'The University Seminar and the Primal Horde: A Study of Formal Behaviour', *British Journal of Sociology*, vol. XVIII, no. 2, pp.135–50.

Home Office (Working Party on Marriage Guidance) (1979), *Marriage Matters*, HMSO, London.

Kanter, Rosabeth Moss (1977), *Men and Women of the Corporation*, Basic Books, New York.

Kelly, Alison (1978), 'Feminism and Research', Paper presented at Women, Education and Research Conference, Loughborough.

Lipman-Blumen, Jean (1976), 'Toward a Homosocial Theory of Sex Roles: An Explanation of the Sex Segregation of Social Institutions' in M. Blaxall and B. Reagan (eds), *Women and the Workplace*, Univeristy of Chicago Press, pp.15-32.

Lukes, Steven (1975), *Émile Durkheim*, Penguin, Harmondsworth.

Lupton, Tom and Wilson, C. Shirley (1959), 'The Social Background and Connections of Top Decision Makers', *Manchester School*, vol. 27. Reprinted in John Urry and John Wakeford (eds), *Power in Britain*, Heinemann, London, pp.185-204.

Mathieu, Nicole-Claude (1977), *Ignored by Some, Denied by Others*, WRRC Publications, London.

Merton, Robert K. (1957), *Social Theory and Social Structure* (rev. ed.), Free Press, Chicago.

Merton, Robert K. (1972), 'Insiders and Outsiders: A Chapter in the Sociology of Knowledge', *American Journal of Sociology*, vol. 78, pp.9-47.

Millett, Kate (1977), *Sexual Politics*, Virago, London.

Mills, C. Wright (1959), *The Power Elite*, Galaxy, New York.

Morgan, D.H.J. (1963), 'Social and Educational Backgrounds of English Diocesan Bishops in the Church of England, 1860-1960, MA Thesis, University of Hull.

Morgan, D.H.J. (1969a), 'Theoretical and Conceptual Problems in the Study of Social Relations at Work: An Analysis of the Differing Definitions of Women's Roles in a Northern Factory', PhD Thesis, University of Manchester.

Morgan, D.H.J. (1969b), 'The Social and Educational Backgrounds of Anglican Bishops — Continuities and Changes', *British Journal of Sociology*, vol. XX, pp.295-310.

Morgan, D.H.J. (1972), 'The British Association Scandal: The Effect of Publicity on a Sociological Investigation', *Sociological Review*, vol. 20. pp.185-206.

Morgan, D.H.J. (1975), 'Autonomy and Negotiation in an Industrial Setting', *Sociology of Work and Occupations*, vol. 2, pp.203-26.

Nicolson, Nigel (ed.) (1975), *The Flight of the Mind: The Letters of Virginia Woolf*, vol. 1, Hogarth Press, London.

Oakley, Ann and Oakley, Robin (1979), 'Sexism in Official Statistics' in J. Irvine, I. Miles and J. Evans (eds), *Demystifying Social Statistics*, Pluto Press, London, pp.172-89.

Overton, John Henry and Wordsworth, Elizabeth (1888), *Christopher Wordsworth, Bishop of Lincoln*, Rivingtons, London.

Roberts, Helen (1978), 'Women and Their Doctors: A Sociological Analysis of Consulting Rates', SSRC Workshop on Qualitative Methodology.

Roy, Donald (1960), 'Banana Time: Job Satisfaction and Informal Interaction', *Human Organisation*, vol. 18, pp.156-68.

Schutz, Alfred (1972), *The Phenomenology of the Social World*, Heinemann, London.

Showalter, Elaine (1978), *A Literature of their Own,* Virago, London.

Silverstein, M. (1975), 'The History of a Short, Unsuccessful Academic Career' in J.H. Pleck and J. Sawyer (eds), *Men and Masculinity,* Prentice Hall, Chicago.

Smith, Roger (1976), 'Sex and Occupational Role on Fleet Street', in D.L. Barker and S. Allen (eds), *Dependence and Exploitation in Work and Marriage,* Longmans, London, pp.70–87.

Stanley, Liz and Wise, Sue (1979), 'Feminist Research, Feminist Consciousness and Experience of Sexism', *Women's Study International Quarterly,* vol. 1, no. 3.

Stanworth, Philip and Giddens, Anthony (eds) (1974), *Elites and Power in British Society,* Cambridge University Press.

Thompson, E.P. (ed.) (1970), *Warwick University Ltd.,* Penguin, Harmondsworth.

Thompson, E.P. (1978), *The Poverty of Theory,* Merlin Press, London.

Urry, John and Wakeford, John (eds) (1973), *Power in Britain,* Heinemann, London.

Whyte, William Foote (1943), *Street Corner Society,* University of Chicago Press.

Willis, Paul (1978), *Learning to Labour,* Saxon House, London.

5

Women in stratification studies[1]

Christine Delphy (Translated by Helen Roberts)

It has been argued that stratification, an area central to sociology, is also an area where the androcentrism of the subject is most entrenched. In a sociology where the issue of class and class structure is central, and in a state within which the breakdown of the population by social class in policy documents, descriptions of the population, and so on is standard, it is clearly an issue of some importance to work from reliable data. At present, the figures on class produced for married women in which it is the husband's *occupation which is relevant can only be of any reliability if we hold the view, along with Parkin (1972), that the family is the primary unit of stratification and that deductions concerning the entire family can be made on the basis of the social class of the male 'head of household'.*

The following two chapters address this problem. Delphy in the light of two French studies, one of which she herself was involved in, and Llewellyn in the light of the British Nuffield Mobility Survey on which she worked.

In this chapter, Delphy points to the inadequacies of present systems of stratification which in the case of women and women alone are predicated upon a marriage relationship rather than occupation. As well as pointing to the anomalies this throws up, Delphy argues that sociology, in adopting this method of classification, actually obscures *a particular mode of production. Thus, she argues, it is not sufficient to see the absence of women from stratification systems as methodological errors or even ideological biases, but this absence is itself an indication of a hidden social structure.*

Over the past ten years, increasing attention has been given to the place of women in social stratification and stratification studies. Watson and Barth (1964) and Archer and Giner (1971, p.14) note that in these studies, the family is considered 'a solidary unit of equivalent valuation' and that the class position of the family is entirely determined by the socio-economic status of the head of the household. Acker (1973, p.937) distinguishes four further assumptions implicit in these studies, of which the most important are:

1   the status of the woman is (assumed to be) equal to that of of her husband, at least in terms of her position in the class structure, because the family is a unit of equivalent evaluation.
2   the fact that women are not equal to men in many ways . . . is irrelevant to the structure of stratification systems.

One might well add that the second assumption concerning 'irrelevance' itself implies on the one hand that wider inequalities have no influence on the (assumed) 'equality' of the couple, and on the other hand that relationships within the couple because they are seen as equal cannot be the cause of wider inequalities. Archer and Giner criticise the fact that the woman's occupation is not taken into account, on the grounds that it contributes to the family income. They therefore retain the family as the unit of stratification.

Acker goes further and criticises first the inconsistency in the practice of classifying a woman by her own occupation so long as she is unmarried and then abandoning this criterion the day she marries; and second, the assumption of the family as a single unit of equivalent status, i.e., its social homogeneity, even when the woman is not in paid employment.

She suggests first that a woman's own occupation should be taken into account whatever her marital status, and second, that the role of women without paid work, i.e., housewives, should be considered an occupation and given a particular place on the occupational scale.

A study of the treatment of women in French analyses of stratification clearly reveals the same sorts of assumption, and in this respect I am in full agreement with the writers quoted above. However, in my opinion it is not sufficient to treat these assumptions as methodological errors or ideological biases which need only be deplored and corrected. I feel that they could well be considered and analysed as so many unintentional indices (as opposed to analyses) of a hidden social structure.

What these writers have done is to draw attention to inconsistencies in the criteria used in the classification of women, and in particular, to the use of a double standard: taking paid work into account for single but not for married women. But they have not examined what this 'inconsistency' itself reveals. It is based on a double standard used in determining social class membership. Occupation, the universal measure of an individual's social class, is in the case of women and women alone, replaced by a completely heterogeneous criterion: marriage.

It follows from this that women are not integrated with a description of social structure through the *application* of rules governing the concept of social stratification, but rather through abandoning these rules. This, in my opinion, constitutes the principal contradiction, and therefore the analysis of this contradiction will be the most fruitful.

The concept of stratification is based on two major premises. First, every modern society consists of hierarchical groups, whether this hierarchy is seen as a dichotomy (marxist theory taken up by non-marxist writers (Bottomore, 1965)), or as a continuous scale (as in American sociology). Second, the principle according to which these groups are ranked and individuals included in them is based on their place in the production process in its fullest sense, i.e., including not only their technical function, but also the relations of production in the marxist sense — status resulting from the combination of both. These three criteria are all combined in occupation, or rather occupation can be analysed according to these three dimensions. It therefore serves as an index for individual categorisation in hierarchically organised socio-economic groups. These are usually further grouped into broader categories for which the term 'class' is used by marxist and non-marxist writers alike.

Thus, we shall use the term occupation to indicate the means of placing an individual in the hierarchy, and classes to indicate the hierarchically organised groups making up the social structures which together form the system of social stratification or the class system. We shall also be using the term 'relations of production' because it explicitly denotes a class system, i.e. a system where occupational groups are regrouped in two broad antagonistic classes in a particular economic formation while the term 'position' denotes a point on a continuum of prestige and income with no sense of antagonism and class struggle. The universal index for classifying individuals and for determining their class position is occupation. It is the only index used to classify individual men, the basic assumption being that all men occupy some sort of place in production. In all modern western societies something like 50 per cent of women 'do not work', that is to say have no paid employment. These women appear in the census as being non-employed. This category is used in studies of economic activity, but not in studies of social stratification.

In what ways, then, do these studies include women, and how are women represented?

P. Naville (in Archer and Giner, 1971) takes the class structure to be synonymous with occupational divisions among the active population, excluding from the class structure any individual without paid work and thus all women in the home. A. Girard (1961) (in *La Réussite sociale en France*) goes further and equates the class structure with occupational divisions among economically active males alone, thus excluding not only individuals without employment and women in the home, but all women. In Naville's work, the active

population is described without being divided by sex, with the
implication that 'economically active' women are on a par
with their male counterparts, whether they are married or
single. But in practice it is normally a woman's marital status
rather than her job which is taken into account. A woman's
own position, that is to say having a job, and one job rather
than another, or not having a job at all, is not taken into account in determining her class membership.

I shall illustrate this by discussing two studies which exem-
plify this practice. One is particularly well known to me, as I
took part in it, and the other is a classic in French social
stratification literature.

The first, whose primary objective was to determine the inherited assets of a sample of self-employed workers, also
sought to measure the social homogeneity of couples and of
siblings, and in particular the relative social mobility of brothers and sisters. The socio-professional categories used were
the ten main categories used by INSEE (the National Institute
for Statistics and Economic Studies) grouped for the purpose
of analysis into three main 'classes'; upper, middle and lower.

The population studied comprised married couples and
included 10 per cent women. Consequently 90 per cent of the
spouses of those studied were women, and 10 per cent men.
The 10 per cent of women included in the study were classified, like the men, in terms of their own occupation. Their
husbands, the 10 per cent of male spouses, were also classified in terms of their own occupations. But the class membership of female spouses was determined by two criteria, which
were not used together, but as alternatives. Employed women
were classified according to their own occupation, while
women who were not employed were classified according to
their husband's occupation.

Other individuals were also classified — the brothers and
sisters of the respondents and the brothers and sisters of the
spouse — with the aim of evaluating the comparative mobility
of individuals within groups of siblings. Brothers of the respondent or of the spouse were classified according to their
occupations. But as far as the sisters were concerned, whether
they were sisters of the respondent or of the spouse, the criterion of classification varied according to whether they were

single or married. Their class position was determined by their occupation if they were single, but by their husband's occupation if they were married.

Two points should be noted from the above; first, all the women in the study were dealt with according to two criteria instead of one in the case of men, but second, all the women in the study were not considered according to the *same* two criteria.

There are, therefore, three problems to be considered; first the dual standard applied to one part of the female population; second the dual standard applied to the other part of the female population, and third the relationship between these two dual standards.

To begin with the last, and perhaps least important, of these problems, what broader view of stratification does this double use of a dual standard point to? That is to say, the comparison of one population classified by two heterogeneous criteria with another population classified by two heterogeneous criteria different from the first two? For the sake of clarity, I shall limit myself to the case of women and their siblings.

Siblings of women in the study: the position (in terms of their own occupation) of women studied is compared to (a) the position of their brothers (in terms of their occupation), (b) the position of their single sisters (in terms of their own occupation), (c) the position by marriage of their married sisters (in terms of the occupation of their husbands).

Siblings of female spouses: the differing social class positions of their brothers and sisters (according to (a), (b) and (c) above), were compared to their own social class position, if they were employed, or if they were not, to their social class position through marriage, i.e. to their husband's social class position.

One might well ask what these social homogeneity rates of siblings and indices of social mobility mean when calculated in this way. A description is as good as its initial definitions, but only so long as one keeps to the same definition. We can only compare like with like and we must avoid combining incompatible categories. But would the study have been valid if the women studied and their spouses on the one hand, and the women who were sisters on the other, had been dealt with consistently? It would not, because in that case, one would have moved from a double dual standard to a single dual standard. In fact, the treatment of sisters comes within the scope of Acker's critique.

Only single women are classified by their own occupation: married women, whether or not they have an occupation, are classified according to their husband's occupation.

On the other hand, female spouses are dealt with in a way which would satisfy Acker since their occupation, if they have one, is taken into account. In fact, Acker's two main criticisms are these: (1) Since many women do not have a man (to give them a social class position) we must consider their own occupation. (2) In this situation it is illogical, having taken occupation into consideration when they were single, not to take it into consideration when they are married.

The implication of this is that if no married woman had an occupation, it would be less problematic, if not perfectly legitimate, to assign a woman to her husband's social class. But from the point of view of consistency, the problem is not solved by taking the occupation of married women into account. Certainly that eliminates *one* of the differences in the way in which the female population is considered: both married women and single women are classified according to their own occupations. But this does not deal with all the problems. Thus, in this study, the population of female spouses (for whom occupation was taken into account) is nevertheless not treated consistently, since some women (with a job) are classified according to their own occupation and others (without a job) are classified according to their husband's.

Thus, not only are female spouses not all classified in the same way, but the whole female population is treated differentially by this use of two criteria, from the population of men, to whom a single criterion, that of their own occupation, is applied.

Since the unit of stratification is taken to be the family, it is not usual to make comparisons between spouses, as this is seen to be unnecessary, and even if it were deemed necessary it would be impossible precisely since, given the dogmatised assumption of homogeneity of status within the family, the social class of the husband is automatically attributed to the wife and there is, therefore, no way to compare social class positions which by definition are identical.

Nevertheless, certain studies are based on this comparison, at least in theory. The concept of homogamy, for example, is by definition a measure of distance — and in particular socio-economic distance — between spouses. In order to proceed with this calculation, it would seem a necessary prerequisite to evaluate the positions to be compared; that of the wife and that of the husband. But even this necessity can be by-passed.

In *Le Choix du conjoint* ('The Choice of Spouse') Alain Girard (1964) looks at homogamy of origin by assessing the distance between the social class of the husband's father and that of the wife's father. But in order to measure homogamy at the time of marriage, that is to say, the gap between the spouses' own social class positions, he compares the class position of the husband with the class position of the wife's *father*. As he himself recognises, 'since social status is defined by occupation, in order to be completely rigorous, one would have to compare the occupations of the spouses'. But, he adds, 'a large number of women do not have a job, or only have one on a temporary basis until marriage. Thus it is *preferable* [Delphy's emphasis] to consider the occupation of their fathers.' One might well ask what 'preferable' means here. Are we to understand that if a characteristic, in this case occupation, is not a good indicator of what we are seeking to measure (in this case a woman's own social class position), we are justified in abandoning this dimension in order to keep the indicator, even if it means changing the population studied (i.e. studying their fathers instead of the women)?

If we are to look at it more closely, however, it is not a case of a methodological error, but a theoretical choice: 'the milieu from which the woman comes being more *significant* [Delphy's emphasis] than her occupation.' But the theory underlying this choice and the criteria according to which the father's occupation is judged 'more significant' are left unexplained. The father's occupation is not 'more significant' for husbands because it is their own occupation that counts.

As far as Alain Girard is concerned, social background for *some* reason is more significant for the woman, whereas for the husband, it is his own occupation which is crucial. This reasoning, whatever it may be, merits discussion, or at least comment. If what is a 'significant' indicator is not the same for women as for men, it is because they are not part of the same system of reference. But there is no justification offered for the choice of different indicators, and no explanation of the reference systems implicitly referred to. On the contrary, in fact, these heterogeneous indices are presented as measuring the same thing. The distance between husband and wife in social class terms is given as the distance between husband and father-in-law.

Not only is the social class distance within the couple not measured, but the choice of indices used prevents any comparison between them. Operationally, the concept of a woman's own position does not exist.

The purported theoretical aim is to study women as members of social groups and as subjects of their relationships. But these groups are *operationally* defined as being made up exclusively of men, and women are *operationally* defined as being mediators and not subjects in social relationships with men.

This problem is not specific to Alain Girard's study. Just as in his study husbands are compared with their fathers-in-law, in the preceding study it was brothers being compared with their brothers-in-law and not their sisters, and in social mobility studies fathers are compared not with their daughters but with their sons-in-law.

These last two sorts of comparison lead us to the most important problem, that of the principles according to which women are included in social groups and the theoretical implications of the criteria used in determining women's class membership. But before discussing this specific point, we must examine the consequences it has for measuring social distance between husband and wife.

The critiques of the treatment of women in stratification studies suggest it is offensive for a woman to be classified according to her husband's occupation, particularly when she has an occupation of her own in so far as this leads to a distortion in possible comparisons between women and between husbands and wives. But as we have seen above, as far as women are concerned, taking their own occupations into account resolves nothing.

The same goes for comparisons between husband and wife, so that in the first study, unlike Alain Girard's, some women were classified according to their own occupations, which allowed us to evaluate their social distance from their husbands.

But all women without employment were put into the same social class as their husbands. The net result is that if, *like her husband*, a woman has an occuption, this distances her from him in terms of social ranking, while if, *unlike her husband*, she is not employed, this brings her closer to him in terms of ranking.

Thus, even when a woman's own occupation is taken into account, putting women who are not employed into their husbands' social class distorts the comparison between the social class position of husband and wife.

In systematically attributing to a woman without an occupation the occupation of her husband, an essential dichotomous variable — that of the presence or absence of economic independence — is obscured. The consequence of this is that a woman who has an occupation, generally of a lower status than that of her husband, is put in a lower social class than the woman with the same husband but without an occupation (and who is, therefore, put in the same social class as her husband). More particularly, a woman who works, generally in a job of lower status than that of her husband, is considered to be more socially distanced from her husband than a woman who does not work outside the home. The fact that a woman is comparable to her husband from the point of view of economic independence distances her from him in sociological terms. Putting a non-employed woman into her husband's social class does not just obscure this fact, it completely reverses its meaning.

What is fundamentally in question, then, in the classification of married women without an occupation and sometimes even with one, is the use of a criterion totally alien to social stratification theory, namely the criterion of association through marriage.

Critics have complained that the occupation of married women is not taken into account. Implicit in this criticism is the assumption of an association between occupation and social class position. If we accept this assumption, we must conclude that individuals without an occupation have no social class position of their own, and are, therefore, neither a part of, nor capable of being a part of the stratification system. But if we cannot bring ourselves to admit that one part of the population has no social existence, we must conclude that not having an occupation in itself constitutes a specific position, which *is* the position of individuals in this situation.

Consequently, the same criticism which is made of the allocation of women who do have an occupation of their own, i.e., the fact that their own occupation is not taken into account, can also be applied to women who do not have a job.

For women who do not have a job, their own social position is not taken into account, i.e. is not treated as an economic situation. Neither is it treated as the absence of a social position, which strictly speaking makes it impossible to classify them with any group. Quite illogically, it is considered as both a necessary and sufficient reason to attribute to them without further examination someone else's social class.

We have seen that the class structure is most frequently equated with the occupational distribution of the economically active male population, or at best, the total economically active population. In the first case no woman, and in the second no housewife is included in this social structure. From an operational point of view then, classes include few or no women.

Nevertheless, it must be admitted by the layperson and the social scientist alike that women, if not actually within the class system, could hardly be anywhere else. The concept of a class system as a stratification system is exhaustive in the sense that it is supposed to cover all the possibilities in a given society. This aim is never challenged even by those who criticise specific features of the concept or the criteria used. Jackson (1968), for example, mentions the problem of categorising the 'dependent sections of the population such as the old, the young and married women'. For him, 'classifying those who are not part of the work force in a stratification system based on industrial occupations presents difficulties.' But apparently he sees these as being purely technical, because although he recognises them, this does not lead him to put forward a stratification system based on criteria which would be applicable to the whole population. Nor does it lead him to challenge the universal claims of a system which is manifestly partial, since on his own admission, it is concerned with only one section of the population.

In the light of this analysis we can draw out several assumptions implicit in the study of social stratification which can be added to those put forward at the beginning: the absence of an occupation is seen to be the same as the absence of a place of one's own in the class structure.

Marriage is considered a valid criterion for determining class membership *only* as far as women are concerned. (No man is classified according to his wife's occupation, even when he has no occupation himself.) This criterion is used over and above that of occupation, even for women who live on their own, since even women who do have an occupation are classified according to their husband's social class.

Marriage brings a woman into the same relations of production as her husband. The determination of class membership through one's own occupation and its determination through marriage are judged to be equivalent. An indirect relationship to class is judged to be equivalent to a direct one.

But if in social reality not having an occupation constitutes a specific situation, even having an indirect relationship in its place constitutes a specific situation on the level of knowledge. This situation characterises women and only women. Thus, it constitutes a sociological class where membership is defined indirectly, as opposed to the sociological class of men where class membership is defined directly. A woman's own position in sociology is to have a place in the stratification system which is mediated and conditioned by a personal relationship.

At the level of knowledge the sociological class reflects and reproduces a social class, just as the position which determines membership of this sociological class reflects and reproduces an actual economic situation. So the relationship of women without an occupation to the economic world is a mediated and not a direct one. Women without an occupation are not a part of the economic sphere whose operation determines the criteria for social stratification, the labour market and the system of industrial wage labour. Nevertheless, they do have a relationship to production, a means of earning a living. But they participate in a mode of production which is not that of classical economics, or rather economics as classically defined. They are neither selling what they produce for money, nor their labour for a wage. Their labour-power is being given in return for maintenance. Thus, not only are they not a concrete part of the labour force, but on a theoretical level too, they are not integrated into the classical mode of production (wage labour, capitalist or socialist). Their specific relationship to production cannot be reduced to the analytical categories derived from classical economics. This relationship is the complementary part of a relationship constituting a specific mode of production, different from and parallel to the wage labour mode.

The existence of this particular mode of production, described by Delphy (1970) as patriarchal, unacknowledged until then, and ignored since, has just started to gain some recognition.

The specific relations of production of married women, whether or not they have a classical relation to production elsewhere, i.e. paid work, are characterised by dependence.

It is this dependence which provides the basis for putting women in the same social class as their husbands. What is more, it is *only* as dependents that women are seen to belong to the social class of their husbands. Having made use of this dependent status to put women in the same social class as their husbands, sociology is anxious to forget this necessary condition and to forget that it is the crucial criterion which allocates a woman to a socio-economic class. It uses it and *must* use it in order to affirm class parity between husband and wife. But having done this, it obscures the premises used, considering only the result, and treats this class parity as a predominant factor in the couple relationship. Or rather, this so-called class parity is used to minimise the dependency relationship within the couple. The relations within the couple, and particularly the relations of economic dependence, are always treated as secondary since the shared social status — seen as more general and therefore carrying more weight in determining an individual's situation — is supposed to override internal disparities. Unfortunately, this 'parity of status' is based *necessarily* and *exclusively* on the women's dependence.

The actual situation is, therefore, the reverse of the one put forward. Not only do the relations of production which put husband and wife into patriarchal and antagonistic classes override commonality of industrial class, since they precede it both chronologically and logically, but they contradict it, since women without an occupation are by definition outside the industrial class system. Certain women, however, insofar as they have an occupation, fall within the confines of the industrial class system. Nevertheless, the fact that their dependence on their husbands is chosen more frequently than their occupation as an index of class membership constitutes a sign, but not the only one, that the patriarchal class system overrides the industrial one.

Thus, the criteria used in determining the class membership of women, if they are analysed correctly, clearly reveal the true position of women. But sociology, by reproducing social reality at the level of knowledge, prevents us *ipso facto* from analysing and clarifying the situation. On the contrary, sociology uses this relationship of dependence in order to situate women within the classical system of stratification. The effect of this is to obscure the fact that women form part of another mode of production. Sociology thus roots its analyses in specific antagonistic relations of production between husband and wife and thus not only denies this relationship, but transforms it into its very opposite: a relationship between equals.

Notes

1   This chapter first appeared in *Femmes, sexisme et société*, ed. Andrée Michel, Presses Universitaires de France, Paris, 1977.

References

Acker Joan (1973), 'Women and social stratification: a case of intellectual sexism', *Americ.n Journal of Sociology*, no. 78, pp.936–45.

Archer, M. Scotford and Giner, Salvador (eds) (1971), *Class, Status and Power*, Weidenfeld & Nicolson, London.

Bottomore, T.B. (1965), *Classes in Modern Society*, Allen & Unwin, London.

Delphy, Christine (1970), 'L'ennemi principal', *Partisans*, November, Maspero, Paris (translated by Diana Leonard as *The Main Enemy: A Materialist Analysis of Women's Oppression*, WRRC publications, London, 1977).

Girard, Alain (1961), *La Réussite sociale en France*, Presses Universitaires de France, Paris.

Girard, Alain (1964), *Le Choix du conjoint*, Presses Universitaires de France, Paris.

Jackson, J.A. (ed.) (1968), *Social Stratification*, Cambridge University Press.

Naville, P. (1971), 'France' in M. Scotford Archer and Salvador Giner, *Class, Status and Power*, Weidenfeld & Nicolson, London.

Parkin, F. (1972), *Class Inequality and Political Order*, Paladin, London.

Watson, Walter, B. and Barth, Ernest A. (1964), 'Questionable Assumptions in the Theory of Social Stratification', *Pacific Sociological Review*, no. 7 (Spring), pp.10–16.

6

Occupational mobility and the use of the comparative method

Catriona Llewellyn

In the previous chapter, Christine Delphy describes some of the methodological, ideological and theoretical problems surrounding the issue of women and stratification. Related to this is the area of occupational mobility and in this chapter Catriona Llewellyn, who was employed with the Oxford Mobility Group, describes work done by herself and Sara Graham while working with the group. Neither this study, which dealt with occupational mobility in England and Wales, nor the Scottish occupational mobility study, included females in their own right in their samples, although the Scottish team did collect information on wives. But as they themselves point out (Payne, Ford and Ulas, 1979) the wives of a random sample of men are not a random sample of women. They exclude single, widowed, divorced or separated women and their selection is dependent on the selection of their partners.

The omission of women from such studies is a serious one, as Blackstone (1980) has pointed out. It is therefore important that such work as has been done on women in this area be published. In 1975 Catriona Llewellyn, working with Sara Graham on the English and Welsh study, undertook a pilot project with the aim of investigating in depth the occupational experience of both men and women in one occupational setting. They felt that previous attemps to analyse mobility data from female respondents had failed to grasp the essence of the sexual dimension they believed to exist in occupational competition. By comparing two groups of workers in the same field, they hoped to highlight and explain in some detail the ways in which sex can affect occupational opportunity.

It is important to bear in mind that at the time of conducting this study the researchers were both employed on two other research projects, and for this reason their pilot study suffered from the constraints of time and locale.

In this chapter Llewellyn suggests that attempts to divide women in terms of two exclusive roles — the domestic and the occupational — are conceptually incorrect and that while the two roles are interdependent, the nature of this interdependency is very complex. She describes a development in occupational mobility research which, although inspired by similar theoretical concerns to previous studies, led to a quite new approach to the study of this aspect of social stratification.

It would appear that because *occupation per se* is used as the prime indicator of class position in mobility research, and broader economic and social relational considerations are omitted, attempts to 'redress the balance' by analyses of female occupational intergenerational mobility, or marital mobility, do not add significantly to an understanding of the class position of women. This is because such studies are still based on the same assumptions of male mobility studies, and the quite different relationship that women have to the occupational structure is never explained.

Occupational mobility research has traditionally played a central role in sociological studies of class stratification. Recent research into occupational mobility has tended to concentrate on refining a well-established approach to the subject through the development of new techniques for the analyses of empirical data. This work has in some cases taken the form of establishing new measures to improve the accuracy of data collected — for example the work of Hope and Goldthorpe (1974) in formulating a new occupational grading scheme. In other instances work has centred on improving techniques of data analysis and on introducing greater conceptual clarity into explanations of observed movement within the occupational structure. Recent work from the Oxford Mobility Group makes a major contribution to this area of study and mobility research continues to be a central area of sociological debate (Goldthorpe and Llewellyn, 1977a, 1977b; Goldthorpe, Payne and Llewellyn, 1978; Goldthorpe, 1980).

However, one aspect of mobility research which is virtually unrepresented is that of women in the occupational structure. As Delphy describes, there have been critiques of the sexist nature of stratification research (Acker, 1973; Roberts, 1979; Steinmetz, 1974; Watson and Barth, 1964) and there is also some American work on female occupational mobility patterns (De Jong, Brawer and Robin, 1971; Tyree and Treas, 1974). An attempt to separate the sex identification characteristics of occupations has also been made (McLaughlin 1978) but few attempts have been made to incorporate women in the population under investigation. One explanation for this is that to include women into such an area of study is to introduce quite new conceptual problems and technical complexities to the analyses of data. Conventional approaches to the study of occupational mobility cannot adequately cope with the quite different relationship of women to the occupational world. For example, the problem of part-time versus full-time workers becomes a much greater one when women are included. So too does the choice of occupational origin for a woman — should we be looking at movements intergenerationally between daughters and their fathers or daughters and their mothers? And what of married women — should we take the occupational role of their husbands into account when assessing their relationship to the occupational structure, to say nothing of their domestic status with respect to numbers of dependent children currently in the household, and periods away from the employed labour force? All these considerations would have a considerable bearing on how to evaluate or interpret a woman's intra-generational occupational mobility. They are known to affect disproportionately the occupational performance of women but exactly how one selects criteria for quantification and analysis is a very much more complex problem, as Delphy has pointed out, than just 'lumping' women into a conventional study of occupational mobility.

If we look outside the limited range of mobility studies, we find that studies concerned with women as employees in their own right have often been confined to studies of women occupationally defined as professional or semi-professional workers (Rapoport and Rapoport, 1971; HMSO, 1971; Etzioni, 1969).

Few studies exist of the occupational stratum where, according to the census, the highest percentage of women in any one group work — that is, in low-level, non-manual, white-collar occupations — mainly clerical and service occupations. Thus, despite the fact that, throughout this century, women, and particularly married women, have formed an increasing proportion of the work force, we are almost entirely ignorant of women's relationship to work, particularly in the sectors where their numbers are increasing. Consequently we are ignorant of their relationship to the occupational structure *in general.* The fact that sociologists have not, in the past, regarded women as an important special case to be considered within the framework of national stratification studies, has not only led to our ignorance of female occupational mobility, but has also meant that female-dominated fields of employment, such as primary school teaching, and other lower professional occupations — nursing, social work, retail distribution and services — have been neglected areas of study amongst students of occupational sociology. If the female labour force is no longer to be seen as playing an insignificant and peripheral role in our economy, approaches to such studies must be made. This work represents one such approach.

Background to the research

The research that is described in this chapter was carried out in 1975 in addition to our full-time work with the Oxford Social Mobility Group. We were, therefore, constrained by two main considerations. The first was time, which limited the scale of the study. The second was locale, which confined it to Oxford.

With these limitations in mind we gave consideration to the conceptual factors which would guide our choice of an appropriate unit of study. Our ultimate decision to conduct the research amongst the staff of the branch of a bank was based on the following considerations.

First, the bank provides employment at the clerical and lower to middle professional levels. These are the sectors in the occupational structure in which a high proportion of women are employed (in 1972, 41.0 per cent of female employees in employment), and the clerical sector is also a growth sector for female employment (21.4 per cent of all 'clerks' in 1911, 69.3 per cent of all 'clerks' in 1966). Such types of occupation also provide considerable opportunity for advancement through a career structure. The 1971 Census showed that 29.1 per cent of all females in employment were 'clerical workers' and (Department of Employment, 1974, p.3):

> In the occupational order XXI, 'clerical workers', the most important occupational unit group was 'clerks and cashiers', who numbered 1,517,200. Of the other unit groups in that order, 'typists, shorthand writers and secretaries' accounted for 737,300 employees and 'office machine operators' for 148,900.

To ascertain differential patterns of career mobility between men and women and the factors associated with these was the primary purpose of the study and consequently the bank, whose employees fall almost entirely into these sectors, seemed to be a particularly appropriate unit of study and one from which we hoped to be able to generalise about a broader group of workers than bank employees.

Second, the branch of a bank is a local organisational sub-system with its own well defined hierarchical structure. Local branches are part of a nationwide bureaucratic system in which policy formulation (amongst which is equal pay and prospects for men and women) and overall control resides with Head Office in London. Instructions on policy are normally communicated from Head Office to branches by means of written circulars. Local branches vary in the amount of business and consequently in the number and grades of their staff. They are connected to the central organization through a system of regional offices (Local Head Offices) which are concerned, in particular, with such matters as control of branch lending, particularly of large amounts, and personnel matters such as staff recruitment and allocation, and the evaluation of the branches' senior staff.

The implications for our study of these organisational features of the bank are, first, that within a branch there is a range of occupational roles at various levels to which, theoretically, both men and women can aspire. In practice, however, in order to acquire a position at one of the higher levels it is often necessary for a staff member to move from one branch to another or from a branch to a Local Head Office or even to Head Office and this, of course, is also likely to involve a move from one locality to another. The decentralised nature of the bank thus highlights one of the problems associated with female upward mobility, namely, the ability to be geographically mobile.

Second, although the ultimate control resides with Head Office the attitudes and values of branch managers may affect the interpretation and implementation of bank policy at the local level. One of the ways in which this was relevant to our study was in the realm of equal opportunities. Although, as we have noted, the bank has an official equal opportunity policy an individual branch manager might, in various ways, encourage or discourage women from achieving career advancement.

The grading system within branch banking

Grading

All non-managerial occupations within a branch are graded from 1-low to 6-high in accordance with a job evaluation scheme negotiated between the bank, staff, staff associations and the unions. It is the grade (within a large branch particularly), which denotes an individual's position within the bank hierarchy. In a small branch with fewer members of staff there would be fewer supervisory posts in, e.g., the Machine Room, and thus it would be possible to see the highly graded occupations in for instance Securities as 'elite' occupations. At the lower grades, the grading of individuals to different occupations is determined largely by length of service, whereas from grade 3 upwards ability is taken into consideration and from grade 4 qualifications. However, considerations of sex also operate from grade 3 on, for where banking exams become a qualification, females are disadvantaged through lack of these qualifications. Many females complained that they were not encouraged, as male staff were, to take banking examinations when they first joined the bank's staff. It is not until after a number of years in employment that the examinations become a consideration for promotion and many females are not expected, and do not expect themselves, to stay in the bank for long.

The system of recruitment and promotion

Recruitment into the bank at the time of this study was the concern of Head Office and Local Head Office and new staff were allocated to branches in accordance with vacancies within a branch and size of branch denoting ease of assimilation of new staff. The Local Head Office recruited largely from schools and some further education colleges and there were no official minimum qualifications, although levels of recruitment varied as regards the bank's employment and staffing situation. The bank had had an equal pay policy for a number of years and a policy of equal opportunity had been emerging. While opportunities were open to males and females equally, until 1974 there was special recruiting literature for males and females separately with respect to careers in banking, as well as separate literature for females such as typists and secretaries and special literature for computer staff. The 1975 careers booklet was, however, for both males and females and stated that 'In banking males and females are equal, with equal opportunities and equal pay. Both can easily progress up the ladder into the management.'

Females and males alike, whatever their educational qualifications, came into the branch as Juniors, but whereas a male employee could expect to go through the Machine Room duties within eighteen months to two years, in practice females could expect to remain in the Machine Room for a number of years. The majority of Machine Room duties are graded from 1 to 3 and so, it follows, the females were at the lower levels of the career structure and the salary structure during this time. The male recruit, however, would be pressured into taking his Institute of Bankers examinations early on in his career (and day release facilities are available to do so), so that by the time he reached a grade 4 position no barriers of qualifications should stand in his way of promotion. Within one department, it was possible to improve substantially on grade level. Thus although no *one* department was considered 'elite' in the sense of the occupations carried out, the grading range of occupations within each department revealed the sort of distinctions, in terms of career opportunities, that exist. Finally, it was part of the bank's policy that all aspects of branch banking be covered and this, on occasions, involved movement between branches within a region. The successful recruit would, then, be one prepared to be completely geographically mobile and here, as I shall expand later, women were particularly disadvantaged. Whilst it is common practice and expectation for a woman to follow her husband wherever his job takes him, it is not equally common, and certainly was not at the time of our research, for a man to accommodate his wife's job moves. This latter point was substantiated by our study.

A number of features of branch banking emerged which, while not necessarily contributing to a *policy* of discrimination towards female staff, nevertheless indicated that inequalities of opportunity existed. We have seen that within a branch, female employees tended to remain at the lower end of the hierarchy while the male employees worked their way up to the top. Although information on methods of recruitment of males and females was scant, we were able to draw some conclusions from the background details of our respondents, and from the staffing attitudes of the bank, that influenced this unequal distribution of labour.

Our analysis of respondents' occupational and educational background revealed that males tended to come from higher occupational origins than females, and that males tended to have higher levels of educational experience and school qualifications than females. The bank recruited staff with their expected length of employment in the bank in view, and it was at this point that recruitment policy seemed to differ as between males and females, for the males were being recruited with an expected length of service of a full-time career, while the females were being recruited with an expected length of service of a much shorter period. The males were selected in view of their management potential and trained and encouraged with this in mind. It was expected, however, that the females would leave work early in their career for domestic reasons, either on marriage or soon after, and with this in mind it was easy to see why the training of highly educated female staff was not an attractive proposition to the banks.

Moreover, according to Head Office Staff Department, in 1974 over 50 per cent of female staff, in all branches of 'High Street Bank', left by the time they were 22 years of age, and a further 40 per cent by the age of 30. Of the remaining 10 per cent — who number around 3,000 employees — many would have commitments of a domestic or geographical nature that would effectively bar them from promotion. In short, the banks would not expect to get a good return on a lengthy training investment.

Because of the mechanisation of much of the banks' routine work, modern banking calls for a core supply of labour to operate the machines and supervise computer terminals. There are, therefore, a number of low-level skills that females can perform in the bank for the duration that it is expected they will stay in work, which require a minimum amount of training and for which the span of the lower level of the grade structure provides a limited career.

'High Street' branch: a case study

It would appear from the following discussion and table that our 'sample' although small, was not unrepresentative of the types and levels of occupations within 'High Street'. The total

number of employees in the branch was 78 of whom 28 were
male and 50 female (23 of whom were married). Our total
sample size, of 39, included just under half of males — 13 —
and just over half of female employees — 26 — (of whom
twelve were married, again just over half of all those in the
branch). The distribution of occupations and grades as between male and female staff was documented for us by the
bank in terms of the different departments within the branch.

Over half the females in the branch (30/50) were in the
Machine Room or Typing section where the majority of occupations are graded 1 to 3 (only one grade 4 and one grade 6);
17/20 of the females in our sample had these types of jobs.
Over half the males in the branch were in Securities (where
grades range from 3 to 5, with one — Principal of Securities —
on Manager's Assistant grade 1) and in Management which
has its own grades of Manager's Assistant, Assistant Manager,
and Manager. In our sample this distribution was similarly
reflected.

Table 6.1 *Distribution of males and females in each depart-*
ment of the branch (numbers in our sample
in brackets)

Department	Male	Female
Management	5 (3)	— (—)
Accountants	2 (2)	9 (—)
Securities	11 (5)	3 (3)
Foreign	3 (2)*	3 (5)
Cashiers	4	5
Machine Room	3 (1)	20 (15)
Typing	—(—)	10 (3)
Total	28 (13)	50 (26)

*Due to ambiguity of titles it was not possible to distinguish within our sample
between different types of cashiers as the bank had done.

Data collection

Our data were obtained by personal interview. The questionnaire we used was divided into two distinct but inter-related

sections. The first dealt with the actual occupational achievement of men and women, linking this to their age, marital status, education and parental background (in terms of mothers' and fathers' occupational status and education). The second enquired into values, attitudes, and expectations. In this section we were particularly interested in the way the bank workers perceived the bank's opportunity structure for men and women and how they saw themselves as fitting into this. We were also concerned with the satisfactions and dissatisfactions offered by the work environment as well as what the employees felt a work environment *should* offer to men and women of different ages and with different home responsibilities. Except for a section of the questionnaire that was directed towards married women, all the questions were put to both men and women and by asking for their views both on their own sex and the other we hoped to find out to what extent norms and expectations about males and females in the field of employment were shared by males and females.

In examining the attitudes and values of the respondents, we used almost entirely open-ended questions. Although we kept strictly to the wording of the questions (this was particularly important since there were two field investigators) we probed a great deal and tried to pursue interesting points and contradictions in attitudes. Since the number of respondents was too small for statistical analysis, we decided to explore attitudes in depth and to turn the interview into a conversation and discussion which was fairly free but at the same time structured by specific questions.

We have already noted that occupational mobility studies have traditionally concentrated on men and when women have been investigated this has normally been in their capacity as the mother, wife, daughter or sister of the male respondent. Although this study is entitled 'Women in the Occupational Structure' it was, in fact, a comparative study. Men and women compete for positions in the same occupational structure but they enter and subsequently compete in it with different sex-linked attributes which consist not just of biological differences but also of different norms and expectations inculcated through an extended socialization process.

We do not, of course, wish to imply that either men or women are homogeneous groups in respect of these latter attributes, but rather that sex is of over-riding importance in seeking to explain different patterns and modes of achievement in the occupational structure in Britain today. The comparative study is, we feel, the most useful tool for explaining these differences.

Analysis

Occupational mobility and banking: looking at the background details

We first looked at the distribution of father's job for both males and females in our sample, as an indication of the occupational background of respondents. Following the work of the Oxford Mobility Group, we looked at the father's job when the respondent was aged 14 since this is seen as a crucial age at which the position of the father in the occupational structure is likely to influence the choice of work or opportunities for the respondent. From our sample of 13 males and 26 females, we found that half the males came from familes where, at age 14, the respondent's father was in a high professional, administrative or managerial occupation. Of the females, however, only 2 came from families where, at age 14, the respondent's father had a similarly high occupation and only a further 7 females came from families where the father had a lower professional, technical or lower managerial occupation. Five of the males came from manual backgrounds, whereas 12 of the females came from manual backgrounds. Despite the differences in sample size, it is evident that, on the whole, the males in the branch came from families where their fathers had a much higher occupation than the fathers of the females. Since it is not unlikely that mothers, as well as fathers, influence their offsprings' choice of work, we included questions on mother's occupation. Choosing the same time/age specific occupation for mothers (i.e. job when respondent was aged 14) we supplemented this question by asking mother's last job if she was not working at this time. (In fact, 8 males had mothers who were not working at this time, and the similar figure for females was 15.) Table 6.2 shows that of occupations currently held, or last occupation, mothers of male respondents were in predominantly clerical and typing occupations (8/13), whereas mothers of female respondents were in predominantly service (9/24) occupations, with equal numbers in non-manual and manual occupations.

Table 6.2 *Mother's occupation at respondent's age 14 (including last occupation if not working)*

	Males	Females
Higher professional	—	—
Lower professional		
(e.g. teacher, nurse, etc.)	—	1
Non-manual clerical and commercial		
(e.g. clerk, typist, secretary)	8	7
Service		
(e.g. shop assistant, cook)	4	9
Manual		
(e.g. assembly, factory work)	1	7
Total	13	24*

* The mothers of two of the females had not held previous occupations.

It would appear from the table that the males in our sample came predominantly from families where their father had a high professional, managerial or administrative occupation and where their mothers had a non-manual, white-collar clerical or commercial occupation. Of the females, on the other hand, almost half came from families where the father was in a manual occupation and their mother was equally likely to have either a clerical or commercial occupation or a service or manual occupation. Thus, it would appear that the females in our study were considerably more inter-generationally upwardly mobile than the males.

The educational attainment of 'High Street' employees

Next we turned to respondents' education to see how type of schooling and level of qualifications was reflected in our sample. The majority of male and female respondents attended ordinary state primary schools, although 3 of the 13 male respondents went to private primary schools, while none of the females did. The type of secondary school, however, was more revealing in illustrating the difference between the backgrounds of male and female respondents. Half our sample of females came from secondary modern schools, while none of the males in our sample went to this type of school. Half of the males in our sample went to grammar school, with a further one-third of males going to direct grant schools and independent schools. For the females, the equivalent proportions were that over one-third went to grammar school, one female respondent went to a direct grant school, and two to an independent school. Overall, then, 11/13 males came from selective secondary schools , while only half the females did — 12/26.

The difference between males and females with respect to type of secondary school is further reflected in the number with different types of examinations. None of the men in the sample had any form of clerical qualifications. Thus, the males tend to come from selective secondary schooling and to enter the bank with O levels (11/13) and some with A levels (5/13). The females tend to come from secondary modern school and grammar schools and to have mainly CSEs (12/26) and O levels (17/26) (only one girl had an A level). The girls were thus of somewhat lower educational achievement than the boys on entry into the bank.

Finally, we looked at the distribution of our respondents over occupations, grades and age, at the time of interview in the bank. At first glance it appeared that the differences in distribution of males and females occupationally might be a function of age. However, a closer look at the career charts revealed that age and length of service in the bank were not reflected equally with regard to positions in the bank between males and females. For example, there were no women under the age of 27 who were Securities Clerks, although the two youngest male Securities Clerks were aged 24 and 21 respectively. The three female Securities Clerks were all grade 3 whereas one male Securities Clerk aged 29 was grade 4 — and there were other younger males with higher grades. However, the most striking feature of this analysis was that only one male (Junior Clerk) had an occupation in the middle range of jobs associated with the Machine Room, whereas the majority of the women worked there. It would seem that the males had experienced far greater intragenerational upward mobility than the females.

The values and attitudes of 'High Street' employees

We attached a good deal of importance in our study to attitudes towards work as possibly influencing the choice of, and performance in, work, given that the attitudes and expectations of others can effect the employment conditions of female employees. We sought to explore the attitudes and expectations of our respondents with respect to their own work experience as well as to that of others. All these questions were asked of men and women alike.

Occupational aspirations

The first series of questions related to respondents' aspirations towards choice of work on leaving school, those of their friends, and of their parents' aspirations for the respondent, together with how respondents felt at the time of the interview about choice of work. Had their attitudes changed as a result of work experience? The responses to this group of questions were as follows.

When asked about the type of work they had wanted to do on leaving school, females revealed much lower occupational ambitions than males. Males tended to name independent professional occupations, e.g. architect, engineer, cartographer, or to express a desire for further education — university — or to go into the armed forces via Sandhurst, Dartmouth, etc. The females, however, tended to be either indecisive or to

name occupations at a lower level than the males, such as
nursing, secretarial, comptometer operator, something to do
with children, etc., as the type of work they had wanted to
do on leaving school. This difference in level of ambitions
between males and females was further reflected in their
current work. The females had largely achieved, in the
bank, their ambitions in the commercial sector, or to have
ended up in banking on the advice of careers officers. Those
who had wanted to enter specific occupations outside banking,
e.g. teaching (2 girls), had not pursued them because they
involved further training, largely away from home, and these
girls did not want to leave home. The males, on the other
hand, had not achieved their higher ambitions because of
largely external factors (e.g. failing eye-sight requirements
for flying, or failing to get into qualifying institutions). In
other words, the males were prevented from following their
preferred choice of work and ended up in banking as a
second choice, a steady, secure job with prospects, whereas
the females either prevented *themselves* from following
preferred occupations (i.e. chose not to satisfy the requirements of training away from home), or entered banking as a
fulfilment of their low-level occupational horizons.

These aspirations of our respondents were further reflected
amongst their peers in answers to the question 'What sort of
work did most of your friends at school want to do when you
were all about to leave school?' The males' friends had either
wanted to pursue professional training or continue with
higher education — the same type of choices that respondents
made. The females' friends had wanted to pursue lower-level
occupations, for example nursing, secretarial, or had remained
clueless, as many of our female respondents had done. This
difference between the level of ambition of males and females
in our sample seems to be further related to the differences
in the background of our male and female respondents.
The high status ambitions of our male respondents are reflected among their school friends which suggests shared norms
in respect of the level and range of opportunities available to
males from such a socio-economic background as our male
respondents. The low status ambitions of our female respondents are similarly reflected amongst their schoolfriends,

suggesting perceptions of a much lower level, and a narrower range, of opportunities available to females from *their* socio-economic background. However, whereas the males in our sample can be considered to be those who failed to meet their own occupational expectations, the females can be considered to be those who succeeded, or in some cases, went beyond their normative occupational expectations, in entering the bank.

(Moreover, the different levels of ambitions of male and female employees can be seen to match well with the staffing needs of the bank. In particular, the low-level ambitions of the females fit well into an organisation where there are numerous tasks of limited skill which, while vital to the smooth running of the branch, are not incorporated into the career structure.)

In response to questions on what types of work respondents particularly did not want to do when leaving school, the differences in perceptions and background of males and females is further evident. Whereas the males talked in terms of the status determinants of job choice, expressing snobbery at 'physical' work, e.g. labouring the females talked of jobs they did not want to do because they denoted boredom and monotony, for example shop work, typing, office and factory work. The female views were, furthermore, largely based on their own experience of Saturday jobs in just these areas of work. When asked whether there was any type of work their parents would have been disappointed if they had chosen, the different backgrounds of male and female respondents is again evident. The males talked in terms of parental snobbery against manual work, dead-end work, or insecure work — any work they considered 'beneath me'. The females talked of their parents' expectations in terms of the better opportunities they felt were available for their daughters as compared with their own occupations. The upward mobility of our female respondents was here most evident in the aspirations of the parents for their daughters to get away from the boring, dirty work (shop work, factory work, that they were in) and to take advantage of their higher educational achievements.

Finally, with respect to attitudes to work in general, we asked respondents what, at the time they were leaving school, they considered the attributes of a 'good job' and second, what they *now* considered the attributes of a good job. Here again the difference in expectations and aspirations in work between males and females was clearly revealed. On leaving school, the males all stressed good pay, security and prospects as the most important attributes of a good job, whereas the females stressed pay, variety, interest and getting on with the people you work with as the most important attributes. From the start the males have a much more instrumental attitude towards work than the females, seeing a job as an avenue to personal success, rather than as do the females, providing a congenial atmosphere in which to work. However, when asked what they saw *now* as constituting the attributes of a good job, the male attitudes had changed somewhat and gave a rather greater emphasis to enjoyment in work and having pleasant people to work with whilst they retain their concern with security, pay and prospects. The females, however, had not changed their attitudes at all since leaving school; they still emphasised variety and change in the tasks involved in work as being important in a good job together with pleasant people to work with. While the females emphasised the variety in work which first attracted them to banking and continued to do so, they still expressed a fear of the monotony and boredom associated with their nearest reference group — the shop assistant and the typist. The males, however, entered the bank for purely instrumental reasons as providing an avenue for advancement and it is only once they have experienced work that they show more interest in their customers and satisfaction in the job. Males never mention variety as an important attribute of a 'good' job and this is probably because the majority of them have responsible jobs and ones that involve a variety of tasks in themselves — they have had no experience of routine work (except as a junior in the bank) and their nearest reference group is the professional or manager.

Attitudes to work in the branch

The next group of questions related more to the work experience of the respondents themselves in that they asked whether the respondents had ever thought of changing their present job to a job outside the bank, and if so, why; what things they liked most about working in a bank; what things they disliked most about working in a bank. The majority of the males said that at some time or other they had thought of changing from the bank — mainly because of the dull work while at the bottom rungs of the career structure — whereas very few of the females had ever thought of changing from bank work even though, as we have seen, they were largely involved in the more routine type of work at the lower end of the structure. Many of the males had made positive attempts to get out of banking but had failed to do so because they could not find a better job, were unqualified for outside, had failed an interview for a new job, lack of courage: 'banking "gets you"— it's very safe', got promotion, etc. Very few of the girls had ever made attempts to leave the bank, even if they had thought of it, because of dissatisfaction with the work. Some got the promotion they were waiting for but others decided to stay because they couldn't be bothered to start from scratch elsewhere — in other words they did not leave largely because of inertia. The girls had personal reasons for not leaving the bank — they liked their colleagues and the social life, and together with the variety and interest of the work these were the things the females stressed when asked about what they most liked about working in a bank. The males, however, stressed a much more client-oriented preference for the work, saying they liked meeting the customers and providing a customer service, and only secondarily referred to their contact with their colleagues. Further the males expressed more concern with the job itself and the work tasks involved than the females who placed greater emphasis on the working environment. This is further reflected in the respondents' dissatisfactions with working in the bank. The males showed concern for the uncertainty and lack of communication about their career chances in the bank, together with the slowness of progression and the level of pay — the instrumental aspects of the job, what it will do for them — whereas the females largely complained about unequal opportunities between males and females and the trouble over promotion at the lower grades, the sometimes inconvenient hours, the holiday arrangements, the bad money, etc., tending to show rather greater interest in their colleagues and the day-to-day conditions of work. The girls, for instance, did not express concern for their long-term career prospects — and tended to see differential promotion rates between males and females as unfairness between individuals at the branch level rather than inequality of career chances between males and females generally.

Ambitions

We next asked respondents how they viewed their future. We asked about ambitions, willingness to accept promotion, and whether there were any changes they would like to see in the bank's policy. With respect to ambitions in their job, over a period of the next five years, the majority of males replied that they did have ambitions, largely to go as far as possible — to senior management. Many mentioned specific positions they would expect to be in. When asked whether fulfilment of these ambitions would depend on anything, they replied that it would depend on their working well; the number of openings/retirements; being in the right place at the right time — keeping your name in 'their' eyes. For the females, half replied that they had no ambitions. Those that did specified higher grades or, for example, from being a typist to becoming a secretary. They said it would depend on vacancies and whether they were still in the bank in five years, that is, many expected to leave and start a family within that time period. All the males said they would accept promotion, but if it meant moving from Oxford a very few said they would not because of the social upheaval; they enjoyed the area; they would only do so if it was a job they particularly wanted. Most of the females said 'Yes' to accepting promotion, but some said it would depend on what sort of promotion it was, and explained that they would not want it if it meant more responsibility, and if it entailed tasks they did not like. Most would not leave Oxford though, because of husband, fiance, didn't want to leave home, didn't want to be told where to go. Some said it would depend on moving house, on the particular job offered, on how far away it was or where to, if husband could move his job. In other words, the females were much less confident about accepting promotion in general (for example, to go into Securities or take a more responsible job — promotion seems to be seen more in terms of a higher grade than a higher job). Furthermore, the majority of females could not satisfy the main prerequisite of the bank for promotion — namely willingness to be geographically mobile.

Finally, in this section, in response to the question 'Are there any particular changes you would like to see in the bank's policy as an employer? Do you have any criticisms at all about your conditions of work?' males tended to criticise the inflexible structure of the bank; they were primarily anxious about uncertainty with regard to their future and concerned about the lack of communication; they also criticised the attitude towards younger males, i.e. the age-specific policy of the bank. The changes that males mentioned that they wanted to see concerned more staff counselling, union recognition, help with lunches and travel, more educational help, and a more informal attitude to dress. For the females, many criticised the policy towards women — unequal chances with men, communications with management — 'could be even better', the screens on the counters, holiday arrangements, the policy towards married v. single girls, inspection of personal finance at the bank, the fact that you have to pay to take the bank examinations. The changes they would like to see included luncheon vouchers, facilities for lunch; a more flexible attitude towards clothes; more perks for women. The females tended to display rather less concern for the fundamental aspects of employment than the males and, although references were made to the unequal treatment of males and females, and married as compared with single women, no specific reference was made to careers. The females did not appear to be as concerned with their long term prospects as the males were.

Attitudes to work: general

We now move on to a series of questions which were intended to elicit the attitudes of respondents towards work in general for different groups of people, in an attempt to see to what extent attitudes towards work for 'typified others' were influenced by attitudes towards an employee's own experience of work. Our first questions were: 'Do you think that a bank is a good place for a young man starting work?' 'What about a young woman starting work?' In response to both these questions male and female respondents expressed shared norms with respect to the suitability of banking for young men and women. For a man, some prefaced their remarks by saying it depends what a young man wants out of life, but generally, a bank was considered a good place for a young man starting work. The bank was seen as providing a reasonably good job, if the young man was prepared to put up with the first few years at the bottom; but a young man could go ahead in the bank if that was the sort of thing he wanted. If he hadn't got very good qualifications it was a good job and banking had the attributes of the 'good' job described when the males were leaving school, that is, the facilities and security. It is not badly paid and there are opportunities for advancement. In other words, a young man can get out of banking the things that the males said they looked for in a 'good' job. The females shared the males' attitudes and added that banking was a good job for a young man if he was willing to travel and take the exams — in other words, the females *recognised* the necessary attributes for a successful career in the bank.

Similarly, males and females thought the bank was a good place for a young girl starting work but for different reasons than for a young man. If a girl was not too ambitious and if she was content to stay at the bottom, the bank provided varied opportunities and the salary was good for a young 'girl'; she could also meet people in banking. Males and females alike, however, admitted that although the opportunities for advancement are there, a 'girl' has to push, to work much harder than a man if she is looking for a career in banking.

The common attitudes expressed here with respect to men and women working in a particular occupational setting, in our case banking, were sustained amongst males and females alike with respect to more general questions on what different people should look for in their work. For example, in answer to the question 'What do you think is a good job for a married man of 40? I mean, what sort of things do you think he should be looking for in his work?' there was a slight difference in emphasis between the different attributes of a job, but all respondents mentioned security, a concern with his pension, interest in his work, prospects of promotion and pay. Most also said that by that age a man should expect to be in a reasonably responsible position — all 'middle-class' assumptions about the 'stage of his career' a man should be in by that age. Similar assumptions were made in response to the question: 'And what about a married woman of say 40, without young children?' While the males recognised that job satisfaction (keeping the mind active) might be important, females emphasised interest as the most important features of work for a woman in this position of this age, but all respondents considered that she would only be working from choice, because her husband would necessarily provide the main financial support for the household — in other words, she could choose any job which she found socially or personally rewarding because she wouldn't be working for the money. Neither males nor females thought that the status of the job was, in the case of a woman over 40, an important consideration. Finally in response to the question: 'What about a young married woman of say 25 to 30 with children at school?' all respondents considered that such a woman could not possibly have a full-time job. All said that she should look for a part-time job with flexible hours (preferably near home) so that she could look after the children when they were not at school. Most considered that money would have to play an important role because this could be the only reason a woman in this situation would work. Job satisfaction was not mentioned at all.

All respondents shared, then, equal estimations about the nature and type of work that men and women should expect. They were, above all, 'middle class' views based on conventional norms concerning the role of men as providers, and women as family-centred workers in our society. There was very little doubt expressed about a man's ability to provide wholly for his family and in fact this was largely because all respondents immediately perceived a married man of 40 to be in a career-structured occupation and probably all considered him to be in a non-manual occupation not unlike their own — this was in spite of the fact that of the married women in the bank some were themselves married to skilled manual workers, for example electricians. The material rewards accruing from the type of occupation that a married man of 40 would have were seen to be adequate to provide comfortably for the needs of his family.

These opinions expressed towards hypothetical individuals only reinforced the impressions we gained of the males and females in our sample. While the males came from, on the whole, higher socio-economic backgrounds than the females, the upwardly mobile aspirations of the females meant that, largely in spite of (or perhaps because of) their parents' experience, they shared with the males conventional 'middle-class' expectations of the role of men and women in the occupational structure. We then looked at opinions expressed specifically towards equality of opportunity and pay between men and women to see whether these impressions were sustained, and whether the opinions expressed among members of our sample were consistent.

Equality of the sexes in work

We considered the views of our respondents on three further questions. First, whether it is right that men and women should have equal pay and opportunity. Second, whether men and women who work in the bank have equal opportunity for advancement, and third, whether men and women are, in the work situation, equally ambitious. In this way, we confronted our respondents with questions specifically concerned with women in employment, and their answers did not widely diverge from the impressions given by responses made previously. First, equal pay and opportunity. The majority of males and all but one of the females agreed in principle with equal pay for equal work, but a number of the males expressed scepticism about whether a woman's contribution could ever equal that of a man. This was expressed in such terms as 'providing it *is* the same work', or 'if a woman's ability/intelligence *is* the same as a man's'. With respect to equal opportunities, most respondents again felt that if a girl wanted a career, she should have equal opportunity to follow one. Again, there was some reluctance amongst both males and females to accept that a woman's performance *can* equal that of a man. Some of the female respondents thought that women should have equal opportunities 'up to a point' and wondered whether women were 'management material'. Many women who appeared to resent inequality at the lower rungs of banking (as it affected them) were, nevertheless, not very happy to see women in management positions and a few expressed a preference for working for a male manager.

We asked respondents whether they thought that, at that time, there were equal opportunities for men and women in banking. Very few indeed thought that there were, but most believed that there was a 'changing philosophy' towards women bank employees, and that opportunities for women at more senior levels were gradually opening up. Many recognised that only very determined and forceful women could get ahead in the bank, that is, women with a particular type of personality, not necessarily required by a man in order for *him* to achieve advancement. It was recognised by many that the attitude towards women in the bank was that a woman must prove herself a *career type*, initially by staying on to an older age than the majority of females. In other words, then, respondents saw an age bar operating, which in practice meant that until a woman had proved a commitment to the job through length of service she was not accepted as a reliable and loyal member of the bank, suitable for advancement to the senior levels. What was expected of a man when he entered the bank at 18 — namely commitment to the bank and expectations of advancement, were not considered likely to exist in a woman until she had stayed in the bank well beyond the age at which she would have been expected to have married.

Most women are expected to leave within a few years and this, it was believed by all respondents, was why they were not treated equally with men. Overwhelmingly, female respondents mentioned that the male staff were pushed on more quickly than the female, and that girls were not encouraged, that they must work harder and longer (and therefore be older) to achieve the same level as men. Most women recognised that the bank as an employer had different expectations for men and women. Men were expected to take the examinations, hence there were different opportunities open to them. The men were on better pay faster, and 'they' would always prefer to put a woman behind a man even if the woman is capable of doing the same work — the excuse being that the women did not have the examinations — but training women is seen as a waste of time.

The bank's inequalities of opportunity are perceived similarly by both male and female employees and the rationale for these inequalities was also understood by both sexes. The majority of males and females appeared to regard the bank's policy towards women as reasonable — the women did not take their resentment very far. Perhaps the most resentful women left for alternative employment — we had no way of knowing. What seemed clear was that the bank's policy was not in conflict with the system of values and expectations held by both the male and female employees. Whether the policy was responsible for values and expectations, or whether the bank could sustain its unequal policy because of the normative system (in terms of sex roles) in which it operated, was not clear, but it was likely that these were mutually reinforcing influences.

The majority of the respondents did not think that women were as ambitious as men in their work. They divided women into two categories: those who were 'career girls' and as ambitious as men (if not more so), and others who saw work as 'filling in' before marriage. Men, however, who knew they had a long career before them, had ambitions early in their careers. Male respondents, particularly, saw an age difference in this respect between men and women, where women only began to have ambitions in their mid-20s, when their emotional lives were 'sorted out'. Young women were not as ambitious as young men because they expected to get married and their main aim was to have a family. They themselves did not expect to work for more than a few years. One girl made the point that in the bank they did not employ ambitious women. They only took school-leavers whom 'they' (the bank) expected to work for a few years — 'It's cheaper for them in the long run'; 'they don't have to train them much', etc. Evidence for this view, from our sample, was seen where some girls who had been in the bank for ten years or so were nowhere like as advanced as men much younger than them. On the whole, however, a self-fulfilling prophecy was evident. The norms for a woman's role were adhered to as much by the women themselves as they were presented by the males.

A summary of this analysis can now be made. In all cases females and males shared the same normative views on the role of men and women in employment and in the family. Men expect and are expected to work for most of their life. Furthermore, men are expected to be the major (if not the only) breadwinner of the family. The type of employment our male respondents chose, then, was one where career prospects gave opportunities for advancement over the years of work in a secure job which implied a continued financial reward. These were seen by males and females alike in our sample to be the major concerns for men in employment, with job satisfaction a desired but secondary feature. Women are expected, and often expect, to confine their energies to their primary role in the family. This role is often not assumed until after marriage and a minimal financial base is established in the home. A woman's relation to the employment structure then is construed as one of a temporary worker whose aim is to acquire the financial rewards necessary to help set up a home and whose career ambitions are minimal. The expectations of only a temporary period in employment influences choice of employment, which our female respondents preferred to involve interesting work in an atmosphere which was socially rewarding. For the exceptional females who remained in employment after their mid-20s, it was apparent that only gradually did their expectations change as to their primary role in life. The realisation that occupation was to continue to be a major focus led these females into taking a more ambitious view of their own occupational role. This, however, was only after their expectations of marriage were seriously called into question by virtue of their age. Marriage and career were never seen as co-existent (for women) either by our respondents or by the bank employers. It is this concept of two types of women then — the career 'girl' and the family-oriented 'girl' — which rendered the belief in equal pay and equal opportunity quite consistent with our female respondents' own work behaviour, and with the opinions expressed on females' ambitions. The career girl is seen as deserving equal opportunities with men and as being as ambitious as men. But because the predominant expectation is that females will leave work at a relatively early age, the career girl must wait until she has satisfied her employer that her intentions are honourable before her occupational commitment is considered seriously. Thus an age-specific policy was assumed in the bank towards single women and promotion.

We must conclude, then, that the inequalities that exist within banking stem from universally held expectations as to the career performance of the majority of females and these are normatively defined and, to some extent, normatively sanctioned. Even where a formal policy of equal opportunity exists, these expectations persist, and lead to inequalities in practice. Many females do not take advantage of the opportunities open to them and employers are happy to let intelligent women carry out low-level tasks for the duration of their employment, and justify their exclusion from management by homilies that reflect women's lack of experience in responsible positions. In short, women seem to need positive discrimination, at least in the form of encouragement, if they are to play full and responsible roles outside the home and to give them the confidence in themselves as an employee group and to exercise their abilities to the full. Only in this way will women begin to bring about a change in the attitudes to female employment that prevail.

It was stated earlier that we recognised the pilot nature of our work both in terms of attempting a new approach to a study of occupational attainment and in terms of the limitations imposed upon our area of empirical investigation. What we would hope to have illustrated, however, are some limitations of a conventional methodological approach and its inability to explain fully one major dimension of inequality in the occupational field. While we are specifically concerned to look at the sexual dimension of inequality in the occupational market, there are of course other dimensions — for example race, religion — which might also benefit from a comparative approach.

We found from our study that occupations did not mean the same *to* men and women, nor *for* men and women. Nor, we must assume, do they mean the same to all men or to all women. These factors, we feel, can only be explained by looking at the complex system of social norms, attitudes and opinions which govern behaviour in the occupational field (as elsewhere). In our study of the employees of a branch bank, we sought to investigate:

1 The occupational experiences of men and women in an occupational setting where, (a) we knew women to be well represented, and (b) equality of opportunity was professed.
2 The attitudes that men and women expressed about their own relationship to their work.
3 The attitudes that men and women expressed to the relationships of other people to work.
4 The attitudes that men and women expressed to equal pay and equal opportunity for women in work.

It is these qualitative aspects of empirical research which we feel have been largely untapped in most mobility research to date. This, together with another traditional shortcoming — the lack of any serious research into women's occupational roles — was what guided our own research undertaking.

The comparative approach described above needs to be developed further, and we hope that future research would both do this, and extend it to a wider field.

References

Acker, Joan (1973), 'Women and Social Stratification: a Case of Intellectual Sexism', *American Journal of Sociology*, vol. 78, pp.936–45.

Blackstone, T. (1980), 'Falling Short of Meritocracy', *Times Higher Educational Supplement*, 18 January, p.14.

Department of Employment, (1974), *Women and Work: a Statistical Survey*, Manpower Paper No. 9, HMSO, London.

De Jong, P.Y., Brawer, M.J. and Robin, S.S. (1971), 'Patterns of Female Intergenerational Mobility: a Comparison with Male Patterns of Intergenerational Mobility', *American Sociological Review*, vol. 36, pp.1033–42.

Etzioni, A. (1969), *The Semi-Professionals and their Organisations*, Free Press, New York.

Goldthorpe, J. (in collaboration with Catriona Llewellyn and Clive Payne) (1980), *Social Mobility and Class Structure in Modern Britain*, Clarendon Press, Oxford.

Goldthorpe, J. and Llewellyn, C. (1977a), 'Class Mobility in Modern Britain: Three Theses Examined', *Sociology*, vol. II, no. 2, May, pp.257–87.

Goldthorpe, J. and Llewellyn, C., (1977b), 'Class Mobility: Intergenerational and Work Life Patterns', *British Journal of Sociology*, vol. 28, no. 3, September, pp.269–302.

Goldthorpe, J., Payne, C. and Llewellyn, C. (1978), 'Trends in Class Mobility', *Sociology*, vol. 12, no. 3, September, pp.441–68.

HMSO (1971), *The Employment of Women in the Civil Service: the Report of a Departmental Committee*.

Hope, K., and Goldthorpe, J. (1974), *The Social Grading of Occupations*, Oxford University Press, London.

McLaughlin, Steven D. (1978), 'Occupational Sex Identification and the Assessment of Female Earnings Inequality', *American Sociological Review*, vol. 43, pp.909–21.

Payne, G., Ford, C. and Ulas, M. (1979), 'Occupational Change and Social Mobility in Scotland Since the First World War', paper presented to British Association for Advancement of Science, Edinburgh, September 1979; (to appear in M. Gaskin (ed.) *The Political Economy of Tolerable Survival*, Croom Helm, London, 1981).

Rapoport, R., and Rapoport, R. (1971), *Dual Career Families*, Penguin, Harmondsworth.

Roberts, H. (1979), 'Women, Social Class and IUD Use', *Women's Studies International Quarterly*, vol. 2, no. 1, pp.49–56.

Steinmetz, Suzanne, K. (1974), 'The Sexual Context of Social Research', *American Sociologist*, vol. 9, no. 3, August, pp.111–16.

Tyree, Andrea and Treas, Judith (1974), 'The Occupational and Marital Mobility of Women', *American Sociological Review*, vol. 39, pp.293–302.

Watson, Walter B. and Barth, Ernest A., (1964), 'Questionable Assumptions in the Theory of Social Stratification', *Pacific Sociological Review*, no. 7, Spring, pp.10–16.

7

The expert's view?[1]

The sociological analysis of graduates' occupational and domestic roles

Diana Woodward and Lynne Chisholm

In common with some other varieties of academic specialist, the sociologist frequently has difficulty in convincing the lay public, including the subjects of her research, that the sociological perspective can provide a special understanding of people's social situation above and beyond that available through common sense. Just as the professionalisation process for occupations in education and social work has been handicapped because 'everybody knows' about education having experienced it themselves, and about social problems through 'knowledge' received via the media, sociological research can suffer similarly from its concern with aspects of everyday life rather than arcane and esoteric activities such as atom-splitting and transplant surgery. Our raw data commonly concern matters immediately accessible to the non-sociologist, and this can pose problems for us in justifying our work as reputable academic endeavour. Attacks on sociologists' work for 'pseudery' or the alleged use of jargon, or for spending time and money to establish what 'everybody' already knew, are examples of the kinds of difficulty we face. These must be overcome if we are to motivate potential research subjects to co-operate and are to secure the necessary approval of research-funding bodies and those who control access to the institutions or groups we hope to study. The extent of this support will partly depend on the degree to which the stated goals of the research and the methods employed to attain them are regarded as important and academically legitimate, and how far the project's staff are judged to be competent and reputable.

These issues may well prove troublesome when the research proposes to deal with an area of supposed common knowledge; or if no hard data-gathering techniques are to be used; if the research staff are predominantly young, female and hence junior in status; and if the focus of the research has a feminist orientation.

In their chapter, Diana Woodward and Lynne Chisholm discuss the way in which a number of these problems emerged in the course of their work on the Second National Survey of 1960 graduates. They describe the extent to which these issues had a bearing on the way in which the work was conducted, the kinds of data collected, and the interpretation of these data. Beginning with a natural history of the project, they go on to outline the problems encountered before finally discussing the way in which the research process may have been affected by a research team which was not only all female (apart from the director), but which was also fully aware of, and sympathetic to, the feminist critique of both the research process and the research product.

The history of the 1960 Graduates Project: the First Survey

The Higher Education Research Unit was established at Sheffield University after Professor Keith Kelsall had been asked to undertake a survey of a specific cohort of university graduates. The request originated from the Statistics Committee of the Secretaries of Universities Appointments Boards in 1964 and it arose from their concern at the scanty information then available on graduates' careers and activities after leaving university. The Department of Education and Science initially funded both this project and one on postgraduates carried out by E. Rudd and S. Hatch (1968) and subsequently a grant was awarded by the Social Science

Research Council. It was decided that the 1960 graduate cohort should be studied on a national basis. This was the first post-war generation to be largely unaffected by the requirement to do National Service, and the interval of six years between their graduation and the study was thought sufficiently lengthy for the study to provide useful information. Twenty thousand men and women had graduated in 1960 — too large a number to survey in view of the wide range of data which it was planned to collect, and so a scaling-down procedure was used to reduce the sample size. Graduates in medicine, dentistry and veterinary science were excluded on account of the extended length and directly vocational nature of their courses, and the senior staff of Bristol University declined to have it included in the survey because, we think, its graduates had recently been studied in connection with another research project. Overseas students and those registered for London University external degrees were also excluded. Since twice as many men as women had graduated in 1960 it was also decided to study all the remaining women graduates but only half the men, giving a final sample size of about 5,000 men and 5,000 women. The Registrars and Appointments Secretaries of the institutions from which they had graduated provided their last known addresses, which were often those of their parents, and the laborious process began of locating the graduates' current whereabouts. In many cases the parents' addresses of 1960 still led directly or indirectly to respondents. Otherwise some success was had with a 'snowball' technique of sending out with the questionnaire lists of fellow graduates so that those whom we were able to trace could help us locate others with whom they had maintained contact (Kelsall, Poole and Kuhn, 1972b). Where we had some information about graduates' probable occupation we could use professional associations' registers of members and other directories (e.g. to trace theology graduates becoming clergymen or law graduates becoming solicitors or barristers), and telephone directories could be used if we knew that graduates or their parents were living in a particular district. Women who had taken their husbands' surnames on marriage were often more difficult to locate than their male peers but this was largely outweighed by their higher propensity to have kept in contact with each other.

Eventually, through herculean efforts being made to locate non-respondents, a response rate of 80 per cent was achieved. The lengthy mailed questionnaire dealt with the graduates' secondary and tertiary education, postgraduate study, work history, own parents' and siblings' education, father's occupation, and — for women respondents only — domestic responsibilities, experience of sex discrimination and voluntary work. The questionnaire booklet had been attractively (but expensively) professionally designed and printed in two colours. A pilot study using some of the half of the men graduates who were not to be included in the survey itself had shown the benefits of this attractive document for the response rate, in comparison with a cheaply-produced duplicated questionnaire.

This data-collection exercise yielded a final harvest of nine 80-column punched cards of information about each of the 8,000 respondents. Not surprisingly, it took several years to process, analyse and write up these findings as only two researchers were employed on the project. Keith Kelsall had originally appointed Anne Poole, recruiting her directly from her first degree, and she was later joined by Annette Kuhn who had just completed her masters degree. Both were Sheffield University sociology graduates. The only further staff for most of the First Survey were Beryl Ibbotson, who was the project's secretary for nine years in all, and a part-time specialist in computing and statistics.[2]

By the early 1970s the survey's main findings had been written up in the form of a monograph, a book and a number of articles dealing with the methodological aspects of the project or with various sub-groups of respondents (Kelsall, Poole and Kuhn 1970, 1971a, 1971b, 1972a, 1972b). Probably because all the Research Unit's staff were women apart from the director, Keith Kelsall (who at that stage received no income from the Unit's funds and was heavily occupied with his professorial and professional duties outside the project), the analyses of the women graduates' situation formed a significant section of the main publication, and much of the public response to the findings was focused on this aspect of the research.

The Second Survey

Having completed work on the First Survey the research team submitted an application for SSRC funds in 1972 to survey a different group of graduates to compare with the 1960 cohort, and the 1970 group was suggested. After the usual lengthy period for preparing and submitting the application and then waiting for it to be assessed by referees and considered by the relevant committees, the SSRC finally turned it down. By this time — as the folklore of the Research Unit has it — the researchers and secretary were sitting with their coats on and the typewriter covered, waiting to hear whether they were about to become unemployed or re-employed. Instead of the proposed new study the SSRC suggested a second survey of the same 1960 graduates to provide a longitudinal analysis of their activities. As the project's existing funding was about to run out, it had become a pressing matter to obtain further finance. A new research proposal in line with the SSRC's suggestions was quickly drawn up and the size of the grant requested was pruned to £50,000. This was less than the sum ideally required, but represented the upper limit for applications to be considered at the next round of meetings of the appropriate SSRC committees. Larger requests would not be considered until after the Research Unit's existing funding had ended. This application was granted.

Thus in January 1973 the Second Survey of the 1960 graduates began, this time funded entirely by the SSRC. Annette Kuhn had left after the First Survey to take up a research post with the University Students' Union. Her place was taken by Diana Woodward who, having just finished her doctorate on women students in male-dominated disciplines, was attracted to the Research Unit by its noted interest in women graduates' situations.

It had been decided that the second questionnaire should go out to as many respondents of the 1966 survey as could be located, and the study would ask for details of respondents' situation in October 1973, exactly seven years after the previous survey and thirteen years since graduation. The layout and design of the 1973 questionnaire proved to be less attractive than the earlier one, due to the constraints of cost and time, after the designer originally approached finally proved unable to do the work in time. Too late to make changes, it was realised that the type-face selected for the 1973 questionnaire by the designer subsequently commissioned to do the job was the same as that used for printed public examination papers. We expected that many graduates would consequently experience negative reactions to our questionnaire, perhaps without realising why.

The process of relocating previous respondents after a seven-year interval was very difficult. As no repeat study of them had been planned the standard of record-keeping was less meticulous than we would have wished, with hindsight. For some respondents we did have recent addresses, as two projects had been done since 1966 by other people using samples drawn from our records of the 1960 graduates. However, as in 1966, a great deal of time, effort and painstaking research had to be put into the process of tracking down respondents using the same kind of techniques as in the First Survey. The snowball list of fellow graduates proved a much less useful technique for locating respondents' peers by this stage, so long after graduation, but eventually through the use of directories, letters to parents and employers mentioned in the 1966 questionnaire, trade unions' and professional associations' lists of members, together with numerous reminder letters, a response rate was obtained of 70 per cent of those who had completed the earlier questionnaire.

The questionnaire responses were coded as they had been in the First Survey by students temporarily employed in their vacation, and were then translated onto a further nine 80-column cards per respondent (making eighteen cards each, for the two surveys), to be processed by computer using SPSS. Major problems in this data-processing stage included human error in the coding and punching of the data, and the sheer difficulty of handling such a large amount of information. The production of the computer tabulations of results was seriously delayed by the size of the program required to deal with all these data. The Sheffield University computing staff operated a system such that large operations like ours were only allowed one run a week on the computer — an opportunity which was wasted if even one comma was out of place in the program or data file. Thus it proved to be many months before any of the tabulations were produced. We felt — we cannot tell with how much justification — that these delays were exacerbated by the marginal status of the part-time married female computer specialist employed on the project at this stage. She had not only arrived to replace the person who had originally designed the computer-processing of the data, needing therefore to familiarise herself with another person's approach and techniques; but also she was clearly not part of the male semi-nocturnal subculture of computer users, and so could not share in their store of accumulated knowledge about the idiosyncracies of the computer system's operation. Both of these problems were exacerbated by her pattern of domestic division of labour, which obliged her to work mainly out-of-office hours and to take sole responsibility for coping with the family's periodic domestic crises. This posed problems for her, for us, and for the unit's feminist ethic.

Staffing remained a problem for the project, due mainly to the shortage of research staff arising from the financial constraints on the study, but also in part caused by the turnover of personnel. This seems to be a perennial problem for fixed-term research projects. Lack of job security obliges research workers to seek permanent jobs elsewere, and these opportunities do not always arise at opportune moments in the research process. Added to this, part-time specialist employees will have divided loyalties almost by definition. The SSRC system of budgeting for specific items, as we understood it to operate then (it has since changed to include inflation-proofing for all major budget items), allowed for the automatic payment of salary increases but the original sum allocated to other budget headings would remain fixed. Thus when postage costs increased considerably beyond the original budget — and this was a major item of expenditure in 1973–5 — we had to defray the extra cost by deferring for a year the appointment of a third research worker. Ann Heath, another Sheffield graduate, was eventually appointed to this job: Anne Poole, who had been working part-time on the

Second Survey, took maternity leave in 1974 and finally left the project altogether, taking her accumulated experience of the research project with her. Fortunately the secretary remained to be a repository of wisdom and authority after Anne Poole's departure and replacement by Lynne Chisholm, yet another Sheffield sociologist.

The interview study

By Spring 1975 it had become evident that the computer processing of the Second Survey data was likely to be a lengthy business which the by now three research workers could do little to expedite. Accordingly we turned our attention to the section of the SSRC application where we had proposed a small interview study to supplement the mailed questionnaire data. From then until the demise of the Research Unit in late 1977 the bulk of our energy and enthusiasm went into this study — not least because we were involved in its progress from the planning stages to data collection and writing up. This was in contrast to the experience we had all had in joining the Unit after the Second Survey had been planned, to work on someone else's ideas. Furthermore our intimate involvement in the interview study gave us much greater confidence than did the postal survey in the relationship between our original theoretical ideas, their operationalisation, and the collection and interpretation of the data.

We had promised the SSRC to use the interview programme to study both a fairly representative cross-section of the graduates and also certain interesting sub-groups, looking at their situation and experience in more detail than is possible in a postal questionnaire survey. This initial promise gave us plenty of flexibility in planning the interview study. We identified an important and appropriate general area to study — the interaction between home and work for both men and women — which we decided to investigate by looking at a sample of the currently married 1960 graduates of either sex, with children; where the husband was employed in one of three occupations which were well represented in the 1960 cohort (namely manager in industry, university lecturer, or teacher in a state school); and, for reasons of economy and practicality, where the families were resident in the South-East of England, the West Midlands or Yorkshire. The particular husbands' occupations chosen were selected not only because there was a reasonable sociological literature on these areas, and considerable numbers of the men graduates were employed in them, with a widespread geographical distribution (unlike, for instance, the location and numbers of pilots or actors), but also because these jobs differ widely in the demands they make upon incumbents and their working conditions. The different types of career and work rhythms would generate a theoretically interesting variation between the jobs in terms of the repercussions of the men's work for their other roles, and conversely, the extent to which their extra-occupational roles impinged upon their work. Thus we could explore the implications of the men's jobs for their families' life styles in general, as well as narrowly comparing the nature of careers in the three occupations.

The three geographical areas were chosen to offer the maximum regional diversity compatible with our resources of womanpower, time and money. As seems to be common practice in this kind of empirical research, an important consideration was the location of relatives or friends who could lodge us cheaply while we were 'on the road'. But within this general constraint we were fairly satisfied with the geographical distribution of the couples interviewed. The South-East had, not surprisingly, the greatest concentration of managers, but as the West Midlands and Yorkshire are areas of considerable size and diversity, with a number of major manufacturing centres and university towns, the distribution of the three occupations was not unduly biased.

The 'interesting sub-groups' of respondents selected for the interview study were a small sample of dual-career families (i.e. where each partner had pursued a professional-level career without interruption) who were married with children; and single women graduates, the study of whom would be Lynne's Ph.D. topic.[3] We wanted to study some dual-career families partly because a considerable if not wholly satisfactory literature existed on this family pattern, but mainly since they represented a tiny minority of the 1960 graduates whose innovatory manner of integrating the demands of two professional-level careers and their domestic roles would provide an illuminating contrast with the other families to be studied. We wanted to know from both the 'conventional' and the 'unusual' couples how they had come to adopt their living pattern, how they managed to integrate potentially conflicting demands, and their ideological justification for their life style.

It was a laborious but fairly straightforward operation to identify respondents who fulfilled our selection criteria and who were willing to be interviewed. This had to be done manually by sorting through the 1973 questionnaires to find those eligible. It had been hoped to use the computer for this operation, but the computing delays made this impossible at the time when we required the selection process to take place. Having identified those eligible, we used a stratified random sampling procedure to select a sample of respondents whom we would approach for interview. After we had done a pilot study of local couples who were eligible but not within the sample selected, to test the interview schedule and to train ourselves to conduct each interview in as similiar a manner as we could achieve, it emerged that our selected interview sample would be far too large for our resources to handle. Our excess of enthusiasm and concern for statistically adequate numbers in each cell, which led to a selection of an excessively large sample, seem to be common faults of inexperienced researchers. The transcription of the taped interviews would alone far exceed the time and budget allocated to this operation, according to the secretary's calculations, quite apart from the time needed to analyse the data. Thus we had to scale down the sample size, using a similar randomised de-selection procedure to the one we had used to select them in the first place.

After six months of intensive travelling and interviewing we finally secured usable interviews with 100 couples plus 6 'dual-career family' couples and 67 single women graduates, i.e. 279 individuals in all, which was almost exactly the number we had planned. The interviews with the couples covered each partner's education and work history, their domestic division of labour (including child care, housework and household financial arrangements), the education of their children, family and personal leisure patterns, and family building and contraception. The single women's interviews dealt with their education, work history, and leisure activities. The interview schedule had been worked out jointly by the three research workers. As we had already decided to conduct the interviews ourselves this collective planning process helped to promote consistency in our interpretation of the questions and administration of the interview as a whole. Although certain differences of approach did subsequently emerge we felt that these were relatively unimportant, compared with the problems associated with the common habit of employing outside agencies, and our own experiences were invaluable in the later analysis of the interview material. Our familiarity with the contents of the interviews and with respondents' situations provided numerous insights which would not necessarily have been evident from the typed transcripts.

As each interview tended to last 1½–2 hours and to yield 20–30 pages of close-typed transcript, we felt amply satisfied with the quantity and quality of the data obtained for this part of the project, particularly in view of our relative inexperience in social research. In retrospect this inexperience was not without its advantages. Although Diana Woodward and Lynne Chisholm had already done some interviews, in both cases this had been for their own small-scale, low-budget postgraduate research projects. But the recent nature of our research training probably inclined us to be far more rigorous and meticulous – possibly to excess – in the planning and execution of this project than cynical, hard-bitten old hands at the research game seem at times to be. We were still concerned to 'do it by the book' rather than being motivated to publish data, however imperfect, and our idealism had not been tainted with the pragmatic concern to get things done by cutting corners.

Analysis and writing up

By early 1976 the interview programme had been completed and transcription of the tapes was going well. However the computer processing of the Second Survey data was making slow progress and it seemed unlikely that this would be finished before our SSRC grant was due to end in December of that year. The problems with the computer operation were the same as always: infrequent runs, mechanical breakdown and delay, human error, and communication difficulties between our specialist and those in charge of the computer system, as well as between herself and the rest of the Research Unit. The research workers conceded the priority of work on the main survey in relation to our 'baby', the interview study, but we were not altogether unhappy about the computing delays. They released us to work almost exclusively on the interpretation and writing up of the interview material, a mammoth task on which we enthusiastically embarked. The transcribed interviews had yielded half a filing cabinet of typed verbatim scripts and although our fairly strict use of the interview schedule meant that specific information was located at consistent points within the interview (e.g. work history first, family planning last) the sheer volume of data made it difficult to know where to start with the analysis of the information. We were fortunate, at this stage, to be invited to present papers at a conference organised by the SSRC Survey Unit (which, like our own unit, was in a state of incipient demise) on the methodological problems of longitudinal studies. The content of the various papers presented there sticks in the mind less than does a happy encounter with researchers from Aberdeen University who had developed a computerised labelling scheme for locating information in interview transcripts. This proved to be a most useful tool for us, enabling quick identification of all references throughout the interviews to whatever items we had thought it worth labelling, as well as providing an at-a-glance record of the topics referred to in each person's interview (see Samphier, 1976, and Chisholm, Heath and Woodward, 1977.)

Apart from two papers written for the SSRC methodology conference and an earlier one based on the First Survey's results (Woodward, 1976; Chisholm, 1976; Woodward, 1974), writing up continued through 1976 and into 1977, made possible by an extension of the SSRC grant given on account of the computing delays.

Gradually the research workers and the secretary left to take other jobs or to do postgraduate study, so that subsequent writing up has been taking place in the interstitial slack times left over from our new jobs. The final closure of the Research Unit forced us very reluctantly to dispose of the completed questionnaires for both surveys. The respondents' written comments had proved a fruitful source of ideas in the past, but they were too bulky to be moved. The dispersal of staff also meant the dispersal of research and other documents, which are now located anything up to 2,000 miles apart, which obviously complicates the process of writing up.

Discussion: females, feminism and the research process

At the beginning of the chapter were listed certain potentially problematic aspects of the research process. Having described the history of the Higher Education Research Unit's activities we can now look more closely at some of these problems as we experienced them. Some of them, as has only subsequently become clear from comparison with other researchers' exeriences, were structural in origin, located in the nature and function of research units in general, and were not in fact attributable to the personalities of those involved to the extent we thought at the time (see Platt, 1976; Bell and Newby, 1977). But other problems were attributable to differences in personality and objectives within the research team. At various times, for example, we had differences of opinion about who should exercise authority over whom and in relation to which aspects of the project. These were demarcation disputes involving all the staff members at one stage or another, in various shifting combinations and alliances. They were resolved either through discussion and more or less amicable agreement (for instance a dispute about how we should respond to an invitation to present a paper at a conference was resolved by us agreeing to give two related but separate papers); or through the disgruntled individual(s) resigning themselves to a situation, having had the satisfaction of expressing their displeasure to the other members of staff; or through successful covert action (for example at one stage the research workers felt that the secretary was exceeding her authority in keeping a record of their time off work, so the offending list was thrown away during her holiday and was never again mentioned).

Yet another set of problems arose from our self-conscious attempt to impose an explicitly feminist perspective on our research, in a field not normally noted for this approach. As mentioned above, the Research Unit's long-standing interest in the situation of the women graduates of 1960 influenced to some extent the interests of the research workers subsequently recruited to the project, although other motives had also influenced our job choice, such as the fear of unemployment and the location of spouse and friends. The Second Survey had been planned before our arrival, mainly by Anne Poole, to gather the same kinds of data as the First Survey, and again with a special section of questions on the married women's integration of work and domestic responsibilities. The interview study then provided an excellent opportunity for us to examine in more detail our feminist-influenced ideas on the situation of middle-class women. We knew from the First Survey results and from our preliminary analysis of the Second that most of our respondents lived conventionally-ordered middle-class lives, had husbands in predictably middle-class occupations and had formed nuclear families. The women graduates were very largely employed in those occupations which had, for various reaons, long been attractive to educated women — mainly teaching and public administration — and they displayed almost universally the pattern of withdrawing temporarily from employment while they had young children at home.

Thus we had to consider carefully how to represent our research to them: a potential conflict existed between our feminist frame of reference and their own sex-differentiated lives, and therefore also presumably between the supportive and rationalising ideologies which they could be expected to hold which would justify their situation, and our own rather different attitudes. Our initial approach to the interviewees was facilitated by their existing familiarity with our research programme. At least one spouse from each couple had already completed the two survey questionnaires, and had indicated their willingness to be interviewed. We could also present the interview study to them, quite accurately and without ideological overtones, as concerning the nature of middle-class family life and, in particular, the interaction between occupational and domestic roles. However it seemed to be neither necessary nor desirable to indicate to them the probable divergence between our own perspectives and those we expected them to hold on issues such as patterns of domestic division of labour and decision-making about employment, leisure, and family finances.

Since we already knew the extent of the sex differences in the graduates' work patterns we wanted to discover whether these were associated with comparable differences in each partner's assumption of responsibility for performing domestic labour, and how the couples perceived and justified their situation. Our expectations were influenced by the studies of housewives by Ann Oakley and others (Gavron, 1966; Oakley, 1974), by studies of housework in various cultures (Dahlstrom, 1967; Fogarty, Rapoport and Rapoport, 1971; Young and Willmott, 1973), and by other studies of middle-class households (Fogarty *et al.*, 1971; Pahl and Pahl, 1972; Young and Wilmott, 1973) as well as by our own feminist beliefs.

These ideas influenced the construction of the interview schedule as we needed to decide how far the experiences of the men and women respondents could usefully be directly compared, using identical questions. Did similar structural opportunities in education and the labour market, norms, values and ideologies, influence their work histories and their performance of family roles? Or would this approach prove not to be useful on account of the fundamentally different nature of the men's and women's experiences — differences which could be explained in terms of the social structural distribution of power and resources, differences in socialisation, dominant ideologies, and so on? In the event we decided to use basically similar sets of questions for the men and women, adding extra questions to the women's interview schedule where appropriate. The two surveys had already set this precedent and we had decided in any case to ask only the wives about family building and contraception. This would avoid the problem of jeopardising our rapport with our older male respondents by asking them about this, and would prevent the duration of the interview with each partner becoming excessive. The extra benefits to be derived from asking each partner about family planning would not, we felt, outweigh the additional costs of doing so. The principle of our not putting exactly the same questions to each partner legitimised our insistence on interviewing each spouse separately and made our investigation look rather less like an attempt to uncover marital disagreement than if we asked them both the same questions (although part of the interview schedule did do this).

Having broadly planned the overall structure of the interview schedule, we then had to plan carefully the wording of specific questions. The common textbook advice is to phrase questions using respondent's vernacular and to fit them to their frame of reference. The problems associated with failure to do this are illustrated by the old courtroom joke:

Judge (to Defendant): 'Have you ever slept with this woman?'
Defendant: 'Not a wink, my Lord.'

But this threatened to conflict with both our feminist perspective and with our desire as good sociologists to uncover some essential truth beneath their accounts of the minutiae of their daily existence. Questions about housework and child care would best fit the respondents' dominant frame of reference if couched in terms of husbands 'helping' their wives, as Young and Willmott's (1973) questions had done. Similarly questions about the wives' work histories would often be quite inappropriate if worded in the same way as those dealing with the men's careers. However, we were reluctant to incorporate these sex-differentiated assumptions into our questions, but it proved a difficult problem, and one which we did not completely satisfactorily resolve, to construct questions which explored just what we wanted to know about respondents' experiences, expectations, motivations and attitudes, but in a neutral and non-ideologically loaded way. We sought to avoid any implication that married middle-class men's careers should take precedence over their wives', or that children's healthy development requires the constant availability of their mothers, which Alice Rossi calls 'the fire-department ideology of child-rearing' (Rossi, 1964). But these were dominant prevailing ideologies for respondents, and informed the way in which they experienced and perceived their own situation.

Some of our efforts to resolve these problems worked quite well. For example, influenced by J. and R. Pahl's book *Managers and their Wives* (1972) we explored the extent to which husbands were prepared (or were not) to subordinate the family's interests to the furtherance of their own careers, and how this was rationalised. Our questions successfully elicited a variety of responses from husbands about this:

'From my point of view the most important thing in my life is (a) the happiness of the family and (b) the well-being of the children — not my career but them.'

'It's not that I don't see my children. I suppose I see them but involvement in them is fairly low because I'm working.'

'Without any doubt it [i.e. promotion] would inevitably alter family life. I should feel sorry if it hampered the interests of the rest of the family but at the same time I suppose as the breadwinner, then this is a thing that has to be accepted really.'

Other questions seem to work less successfully, particularly those where certain key words or phrases such as 'housewife' and 'working mother' triggered off strong ideological reactions rather than a slower, more considered response. The question 'How do you feel about working mothers?' was, for example, only answered in terms of children's alleged needs and not mothers', except by the dual-career wives and the only three wives (out of 100) who were employed full-time and were highly committed to their work. The question on the women's identity as housewives which we derived from Ann Oakley's work brought forth a particularly powerful and emotional response: 'When you fill in a form and write "Occupation: housewife" how do you feel about that?' Two dual-career wives, for example, replied:

> 'I don't think of myself as a housewife in any sense whatsoever. I've opted out of running my house in favour of having a job.'

> 'As for being a housewife, I've never regarded myself as such. He always said he didn't marry me to get a house-keeper.'

The full-time housewives' comments also indicated their awareness of the low public esteem in which the role of house-wife is held, either by repudiating this estimation of their own worth or by accepting it:

> 'I think it's a very important role, being a housewife. You have so much to see to, to keep your husband's life running as smoothly as possible, and bringing up the children so that they're well adjusted to life. I think this is the most important thing. I'm not unhappy being a housewife at all.'

> 'Degraded — in my mind I don't feel like a housewife and I don't like the idea of people thinking "Oh, you're just a housewife." '

Apart from the benefits for the interview study of the respondents' familiarity with the Unit's work, and the problem of our concern to avoid using a sexist frame of reference for the interview questions, a further major issue at the interview stage was our presentation of self (selves?) to the interview respondents. We were open to relatively accurate categorisation as young, junior, female research workers who (as they were often quick to establish) did not have children, and only one of us was married. And as academics we could be easily stereotyped in terms of our probable life styles, norms and values. Thus not only could we have little insight into large areas of our respondents' experiences — areas about which we were interviewing them — because of their age, occupational status and social status as parents, but furthermore by being engaged in full-time academic careers we represented a 'choice' which many of the women respondents had opted to repudiate. How could we be expected to empathise with their accounts of the conflicts generated by marriage, parenthood and employment? How could we understand and share the Bowlby-influenced ideologies of sex roles and parenthood which had encouraged them to give priority to their maternal role over their work role? The very nature of our questions about employment and the domestic division of labour served to reveal our preoccupation with work, marital conflict and women's oppression, rather than with the satisfactions of motherhood and housewifery. The questions inviting respondents to tell us about their children's education, family leisure activities and family planning may have gone some way to redress this impression however.

Apart from trying to word questions in an ideologically neutral way there seemed little action which we could take to deal with this potential difficulty. The problem of establishing rapport between interviewer and respondent is clearly crucial to the success of the research endeavour in motivating the respondent to co-operate. However the methodological problem of over-rapport has also been recognised — the influence on their answers of respondents' desire to provide the interviewer with the material she is thought to be seeking and to secure her approval. In the event our data collection enterprise seemed not to suffer unduly from the effects of respondents' assessment of the divergence between our attitudes and their own; and indeed the very difference between their situation and our own carried some advantages. The balance of status and authority between them and ourselves favoured them by virtue of their greater age and higher social status, which gave them sufficient self-confidence to find no threat or implied criticism in our questions. And the difference between our situation and theirs made it appropriate for them to articulate in considerable detail the nature of their daily lives in a much more explicit, and hence to us useful way than would have been appropriate had we established a wider basis of common experience and understanding. In this, our experience differed from that of Ann Oakley in her study of motherhood, since this was something of which she herself had personal experience.

The reverse side of the coin — the disadvantages of the discrepancy in age, status and, for the men respondents, the difference of sex between ourselves and them — was that a small number of the men treated us with lack of consideration. In some cases they broke appointments without notifying us, causing us wasted journeys; or kept us waiting despite our having agreed mutually convenient times for the interview, and then failed to explain or excuse the delay; or occasionally we were subjected to a rather patronising manner. But on the whole the respondents were extremely co-operative, helpful and hospitable to us. We attribute this to their pre-existing favourable orientation to the research project, and to their own preoccupation with the issues about which we wanted to interview them.

These were the main ways in which our desire to adopt a feminist frame of reference for the research led us to consider some perennial methodological problems in a new light. In other respects our common commitment to feminism exempted us from certain kinds of potential difficulty and enhanced our job satisfaction. Keith Kelsall had adopted a non-directive role as director of the project, leaving us with considerable freedom to do our work as we felt appropriate. Not being subject to the exercise of power derived from rank, the research team could operate in an open and democratic way and, unlike many researchers on temporary contracts, we did not feel that our efforts were being appropriated to promote Keith's career (and this was not just because he had already attained the status of one of sociology's elder statesmen). Since we did function fairly autonomously, however, and in general attended seminars and conferences without Keith, we were displeased to hear ourselves referred to as 'Keith's little helpers', and slightly resented references to the project as 'Kelsall's work', but these were minor irritants rather than the major issues which they have been in some projects. Jackie West, for example, has written:

The assumption persists that where women have participated in research along with a man, it is he who must
have been the effective director of the project (whether
formally so or not) and that correspondingly women
research workers cannot have been equal contributors
let alone partners (unpublished paper on file at the
Women's Research and Resources Centre, dated 1977).

We felt relatively favourably placed as far as the issue of
authorship went in that the interview study, which was
likely to produce the first major publications from the project, was clearly all our own work. However, this independent
effort carries the disadvantage that without a 'big name' or
an author with a good record of publications on the title
page it seems much more difficult to interest publishers.

In some respects the Research Unit as a whole functioned
as a consciousness-raising group. Our ideas were mutually
reinforced by each other as well as by the nature of our
reading, interviewing and analysis, and certain explicit norms
developed within the Unit about the non-exploitation of other
people. When Beryl Ibbotson left the Unit and secretarial
work to become an Accommodation Officer – a much more
challenging, interesting and rewarding career – and when her
replacement subsequently became a sociology student, it
pleased us to feel that our encouragement of their abilities
was in some small way responsible for their changes of
direction. But our missionary zeal was not always well
received: one of the University Accommodation Officers,
who worked in the same building as us, did not react favourably to our criticism of his sexist and offensive language.
This problem, and others, seemed to arise from our anoma-
lous and marginal position within the University, which was
compounded by our lowly status as junior female researchers
on short-term contracts (and of course the majority of such
workers are women). On a number of occasions we had
difficulty in gaining the University's approval to appoint
research workers to an appropriately·high point on the salary
scale, but this situation improved once the Association of
University Teachers had a special salary scale nationally
adopted for research workers, linked to the lecturers' pay

scale and graded by qualifications and experience. We also
had problems in getting formal recognition of appropriate
statuses for ourselves elsewhere in the University, for example
to get listed as 'Independent Research Workers' in the Staff
Handbook and to be allowed to join the Senior Common
Room. This was not just a trivial issue about where we could
eat lunch, but had implications for our representation on
various bodies and networks of contacts. Other women
researchers we know of have had similar difficulties in securing
the payment of annual increments, or in getting their postgraduate fees paid from their research grants. This political
marginality of status is often exacerbated, and was in our case,
by geographical isolation. We were located so far from the
sociology department that we rarely met other members of
staff and we felt excluded from what went on there. After
one department party we were told, 'We were sorry that you
couldn't be invited but we had to draw the line somewhere.'

A further set of problems arose from the way in which
SSRC research grants are organised. Reference has already
been made to the difficulty of catering for all contingencies
within the initial budgeting of the research application. The
inflexibility of the system, and the cumbersome process of
having changes approved by the SSRC Secretariat (at that
time, anyway) promoted entrepreneurial initiative. Fortunately we had been able to economise on the money allocated to interviewing expenses by staying with friends
and relatives and by being frugal. Thus we were later able,
probably illegitimately, to draw on the money remaining
under this budget heading to pay for subsistence of other
kinds, mainly our attendance at conferences and meetings,
when the money properly allocated to that heading had been
spent.

Concluding reflections

Apart from a number of papers on methodological aspects of
the surveys and the interview study, we have given or published papers on the family planning data, on the single
women's careers compared with the men's, and on the

interaction between home and work, comparing the men, the women employed full-time and the dual-career wives. The rest of the interview data have been written up but not yet published, and when that does happen we will write up the Second Survey data. As publishers have been quick to point out, this field of research — an investigation into the situation of a relatively privileged group — is not a fashionable one. The middle-class book-buying public is allegedly unwilling to purchase books about other middle-class people, and our work also lies outside mainstream feminist sociology which is presently focused on general theoretical issues or on less privileged groups of women.

From the interview data we have concluded that these women clearly are privileged in relation to others: their education, work experience and family incomes enable them to exercise their own discretion in various areas of their lives to a greater extent than can most women. In the field of planning their children, for example, they are well informed about specific contraceptive techniques, and are not inhibited from seeking the help of the medical profession. It is not surprising, then, that they are much less likely to become unintentionally pregnant than are women of other social classes and who are less highly educated (Woodward, Heath and Chisholm, 1977). They feel able to make 'choices' about their employment, their children's education and their leisure activities. However, their expectations that life can be manipulated to accord with their wishes are to some extent constrained by their structural and ideological situation. Here their position is not so dissimilar in absolute terms from that of less advantaged women, even if it does differ in terms of the material resources to which they have access. At work, for example, our women respondents may generally occupy more exalted, better paid positions than most women but they are still subject to the operation of the dual labour market (Barron and Norris, 1976). In comparison to the men respondents they are concentrated in the least desirable, lowest-status levels of the least prestigious professions, often work in jobs considerably inferior to those commensurate with their experience and qualifications, and fare worse than their male peers in terms of salary and promotion. (This applies to the single women graduates as well as the wives; Chisholm and Woodward, 1979.)

Like other women our respondents have had experiences of sex-role socialisation, the education system and the job market which have encouraged them to develop less market-able skills than men, and to perceive their disadvantaged situation as broadly legitimate and appropriate. Within the home both husbands and wives independently reported to us a highly unequal division of labour (irrespective of the wife's work situation) in relation to child care, housework and financial arrangements. The dominant pattern was for husbands to decide unilaterally what tasks they were pre-pared to perform and to perceive this as 'help' given to their wives, who faced the choice of colluding in this arrangement or of complaining rather ineffectually about it. However, as their present situation was seen as freely chosen, whereas we perceived it in terms of male dominance arising from their superior economic power, reinforced by sex-differentiated ideologies, the women were prevented from identifying the cause of their dissatisfaction. As one expressed it:

'I miss working very much. I had a far better opinion of myself when I was working than I have now. . . . I think sometimes I ought to appreciate the fact that it's nice not to have to get up in the morning. If I want to spend an hour just reading the paper instead of getting on with something, I can do it now. But I feel that's just com-pensating me for something else I'd rather be doing.'

'Before you became a wife and mother did you have much idea what it would be like?'
'Not really, no. I don't think I'd have realised even if I had thought deeply about it.'

'What do you feel about the way being a wife and mother has actually turned out?'
'I get very annoyed sometimes. I feel as if nature has cheated me. That's difficult, isn't it? I get to the point where I think I was educated to have a career and now I can't use it. And whatever I go back into, I'm 36 now —

I'm not going to make a career of any real kind, and I feel cheated. But I can't think of anybody who cheated me, I did it myself. I can't blame my husband — it wasn't him. I can't blame my parents — they did their best for me, educated me, I'd feel just as frustrated if I hadn't been. I feel that someone along the line has cheated me, something has gone wrong in my life but I can't put my finger on what, or how it could be altered.'

'What about being a housewife, as opposed to being a wife and mother?'
'Well, I hate housework — the monotony I suppose. But I'm one of those people who have to do it. I can't live in a mess, I've got to have the house clean.'

The women's situation must be viewed within its wider social context: society's structural arrangements and dominant ideologies support the status quo and exacerbate the difficulties faced by couples and women alone who seek to move outside traditional living patterns. In this chapter we have been exploring our experience of seeking to apply a feminist perspective to the analysis of middle-class family life, but the realities of the research process are of course far muddier and more confused than this bald statement implies. No single unitary 'feminist perspective' can be (a) identified and then (b) applied in the research situation. Rather, we had a certain imperfectly articulated view of society and how it operates and changes. Parts of this view were implicit rather than explicit, the view changed and developed according to what we had been reading or our own experiences, and we by no means always agreed in attitude or perception. Nevertheless we shared a fundamentally similar approach to this work and hope that this account of its problems, failures and minor achievements will help others to put their own difficulties in context, as we ourselves have benefited from reading the honest accounts of others' experiences of doing empirical research.

Notes

1   The label 'The Expert' was coined by undergraduate friends to describe the role adopted by some men spectators at football matches in providing everyone within earshot with a loud running commentary on the game, consisting mainly of their advice to players, team managers, referee and linesmen, on what they should be doing or are doing wrongly, throughout the game, embellished with the currently popular footballing clichés of the professional commentators.

2   There were — consecutively — three computer specialists working on the project. All were part-timers and all were women with children. They were Corgi Law, Linda Anderson and Christine Hopkinson.

3   In fact, these data were not subsequently written up as a doctoral thesis due to the common problems of the difficulty of obtaining registration for a higher degree as a staff member on an externally funded research contract, and the pressure of work both on our own project and in subsequent temporary academic appointments.

References

Barron, R.D. and Norris, G.M. (1976), 'Sexual Division in the Labour Market' in D.L. Barker and S. Allen (eds), *Dependence and Exploitation in Work and Marriage*, Longman, London.

Bell, C. and Newby, H. (eds) (1977), *Doing Sociological Research*, Allen & Unwin, London.

Chisholm, L. (1976), 'A Small-scale Interview Study Within the Context of a Large-scale Longitudinal Questionnaire Survey', paper given to SSRC Survey Unit Seminar on the Methodology of Longitudinal Surveys, Cambridge.

Chisholm, L., Heath, A. and Woodward, D. (1977), 'Methodological Problems of Quantitative and Qualitative Research: The National Survey of 1960 Graduates', *Angewandte Sozialforschung*, vol. 5, no. 1, pp.195–208.

Chisholm, L. and Woodward, D. (1979) 'The Progress and Experiences of Women Graduates in the Labour Market' in R. Deem (ed.), *Women and Education: A Reader*, Routledge & Kegan Paul, London.

Dahlstrom, E. (ed.) (1967), *The Changing Roles of Men and Women*, Duckworth, London.

Fogarty, M., Rapoport, R. and Rapoport, R. (1971), *Sex, Career and Family*, Allen & Unwin, London.

Gavron, H. (1966), *The Captive Wife: Conflicts of Housebound Mothers*, Routledge & Kegan Paul, London.

Kelsall, R.K., Poole, A. and Kuhn, A. (1970), *Six Years After*, Sheffield, Higher Education Research Unit.

Kelsall, R.K., Poole, A. and Kuhn, A. (1971a), 'Marriage and Family Building Patterns of University Graduates', *Journal of Biosocial Science,* vol. 3, pp.281–7.

Kelsall, R.K., Poole, A. and Kuhn, A. (1971b), 'The Young Science Graduate', *Universities Quarterly,* vol. 25, pp.353–68.

Kelsall, R.K., Poole, A. and Kuhn, A. (1972a), *Graduates: The Sociology of an Elite,* Methuen, London.

Kelsall, R.K., Poole, A. and Kuhn, A. (1972b), 'The Questionnaire in a Sociological Research Project', *British Journal of Sociology,* vol. 23, pp. 344–57.

Oakley, A. (1974), *The Sociology of Housework,* Martin Robertson, London.

Pahl, J. and Pahl, R. (1972), *Managers and their Wives: A Study of Career and Family Relationships in the Middle Class,* Penguin, Harmondsworth.

Platt, J. (1976), *Realities of Social Research: An Empirical Study of British Sociologists,* University of Sussex Press, London.

Rossi, A. (1964), 'A Good Woman is Hard to Find', *TransAction,* vol. 1, pp.20–3.

Rudd, E. and Hatch, S. (1968), *Graduate Study and After,* Weidenfeld & Nicolson, London.

Samphier, M. (1976), *A Data Indexing Scheme,* Aberdeen, MRC Research Unit, University of Aberdeen.

Woodward, D. (1974), 'The Implications of Sex for the Life-styles of Graduates', paper presented to Annual Conference of the British Sociological Assocation, Aberdeen.

Woodward, D. (1976), 'Representativeness and Error in Longitudinal Surveys', paper given to SSRC Survey Unit Seminar on the Methodology of Longitudinal Surveys, Cambridge.

Woodward, D., Heath, A. and Chisholm, L. (1977) 'Patterns of Family Building and Contraception Use of Middle-class Couples', *Journal of Biosocial Science,* vol. 10, pp.39–58.

Young, M. and Willmott, P. (1973), *The Symmetrical Family: A Study of Work and Leisure in the London Region,* Routledge & Kegan Paul, London.

8

The gatekeepers: a feminist critique of academic publishing

Dale Spender

We tend to see one of the ends of research (or in some cases one of the means to an end) as being publication. But little has been written on the processes which are instrumental in determining that research gets reported, or published. It is therefore fitting that the final contribution to this collection should comment on some aspects of the publication process. In keeping with a feminist tradition, Dale Spender uses her experience as a journal editor and series editor to talk about the process of publishing, an issue raised as a problem by Diana Woodward and Lynne Chisholm in their chapter.

In her chapter, Dale Spender looks at some aspects of the significance of publishing and its practices in the research community. Not only, she suggests, is there an absence of 'hard data' on this subject, there is an absence of 'soft data' as well. Indeed, we need an explanation of why so much about publishing has been taken for granted. Kuhn (1975) in his analysis of the personal and social forces which shape the knowledge we construct and disseminate, does not have the process of publishing on his agenda, a surprising omission, but one which indicates that much of our analysis of the way in which disciplinary paradigms are shaped and changed begins with the printed word, rather than with the processes that lead to it. The same could be said of feminism, for while feminists have been acutely conscious of the political dimensions in the construction of knowledge, they have often stopped where the printed word begins. This is to some extent understandable, for it is extremely difficult to gather data on what is submitted to editors, as distinct from what is published. But in the attempt to document the biases that have been encoded against women in the traditional literature it is short-sighted to confine data to published *sources. While influential, the locus of control is not always after publication.*

Spender argues in her chapter that those who make decisions on what does and what does not get published have an active role in shaping a discipline or area and thus raises legitimate cause for concern for those attempting to work in ways which challenge mainstream orthodoxies.

As Dorothy Smith (1978) has pointed out, there are *gatekeepers* in the academic community. These are the people who set the standards, produce the social knowledge, monitor what is admitted to the systems of distribution, and decree the innovations in thought, or knowledge, or values (p.287). Many of these people are to be found as editors of journals, as referees or reviewers, or as advisors to publishers. They are in a position to determine what gets published and what does not, and most of them are men.

In this context, there are four broad areas that I would like to examine. First, I would like to discuss the significance of publication in the academic community, and the – often unexplored – attitudes towards it. Second, I will raise the issue of the role played by publications in shaping a discipline, in determining the 'fashionable' questions – and answers – which set the parameters in which individuals are encouraged to work, if they wish to be at the centre of the issues in their discipline. Third, I will look at the criteria used for determining 'scholarly excellence' and because of the absence of much readily accessible data, I will draw on some of my own experiences in this area. And finally, I will be arguing that when it is mostly men who are in the position to decide what gets published and what does not, there is a problem of male dominance, which demands feminist attention.

The significance of publishing

It is important to make explicit the significance of publishing in the research community. In a very fundamental sense, research which is not in print does not exist. The familiar dichotomy of public and private — with all its concomitant inequalities — is often seen in operation. Few findings are conveyed in their final form by word of mouth, and if they are, they are generally perceived as unreliable. Even references in published sources which contain the terms 'private communication' do not seem to carry the same weight as those that have been printed[1] and without venturing into a discussion of the politics of the printed word, it appears that some mysterious transformation occurs when the private becomes public and personal opinions are translated into print.

There frequently seems to be an assumption that with publication comes legitimation, and that personal opinions, interpretations and conclusions move closer towards 'truth' and credibility when they are contained between the covers of a respectable academic journal or book. It is not usually enough within the academic community to substantiate a case by referring to the work of one's friends, unless it is in print. Granting such weight to the printed word — and placing one's faith in editors to sort the 'good' from the 'bad' — can make the academic community extremely vulnerable.

Not all publications, of course, carry the same weight. Without reference to the contents, judgments about the reliability of a particular piece of work may be made on the basis of the place occupied by particular publishers in the academic publishing hierarchy. This can lead in turn to a hierarchy of publications in terms of tenure or promotion. Such ranking of publishers has not escaped feminist attention (see June Arnold, 1976) for it is sometimes the source of a dilemma. A feminist might have a manuscript that is actively sought after by a prestigious academic publisher, but wish to place it with a feminist press. In this case, she may find that while the manuscript could be an impressive item on her publication record with an academic publisher, it could well be 'discounted' with a feminist publisher.

If it is believed that reputable publishers produce more reliable books because they have more rigorous and rational processes of selection, such a belief could well be misguided. In her survey of what gets published and what does not, Lou Buchan (1980) began with the hypothesis that there was no rational basis for distinguishing between the 'accepted' and the 'rejected', and after two years of research she has found no evidence which would cause her to modify that hypothesis.

Indeed, it could be argued that small, radical, left and feminist presses (which are often the ones to be discounted) are sometimes even more selective in what they publish. Some feminist publishing houses, for example, apart from receiving numerous unsolicited manuscripts (which might not make their way to academic publishers) also operate collectively, and here the manuscript can be the object of close scrutiny, because it is unlikely that those making decisions would be able to comment on the accuracy or adequacy of individual tion were to be given to *all* manuscripts in academic publishing houses, not just because of the time and care required, but because it is likely that those making decisions would be able to comment on the accuracy or adequacy of individual academic manuscripts. Kuhn (1975) comments on this, pointing out that 'learned' communications have moved from addressing the general, interested reader and that there has been an evolution in linguistic style as well as an evolution in scientific knowledge, with research communiqués changing 'in ways whose evolution has been too little studied but whose modern end products are obvious to all and oppressive to many' (Kuhn, 1975, p.20).

Academic publishers will frequently rely on 'experts' as 'objective reviewers' (I will return to this later) who are paid a (small) fee to gauge not only whether the manuscript is 'good' or 'credible' but also whether it will sell. When it is realised that a report which states that the manuscript is 'excellent, but would not appear to have wide appeal' leads to rejection more frequently than a report which states 'inexcusably poor but could prove to be popular' then we can see that the practice of automatically equating reliability with any particular publisher could be misguided.

Because they are more frequently purchased by subscription, journals are not usually subject to quite the same restrictions as books. The question of whether an individual article will be a 'best seller' does not normally arise. Indeed, editors may seek security and status by disclaiming any knowledge of the 'commercial' side of the operation. But we cannot assume that the removal of commercial considerations ensures a more rational basis for determining the material that appears between the covers.

Shaping the discipline

What gets published can influence those who read *and* those who write. While from an academic point of view the emphasis may be given to publishing, rather than to reading what others publish (for it is publish or perish, not read or perish) there can be little question that the 'literature' is instrumental in establishing the issues in a discipline. It constitutes the parameters in which discussion occurs and defines the terms of the debate. But the material that is published does not always reflect genuine concern for the advancement of knowledge.

For what is published can also set the style for those seeking publication. Although it may not be customary, a lecturer who insisted that his postgraduate students undertake an analysis of relevant journals to determine what 'topics were favoured and from what perspective, what length and language was preferred, and so on, was considered to be an excellent advisor by his students who claimed that he had helped them 'crack the code' of publishing. Their stance may have been considered cynical by some, for after the students had decided what was required, they proceeded to tailor-make their research to fit it. While they achieved excellent publication records, which were no liability in their careers, their expertise sometimes lay in producing what was wanted (and there are many implications of this) and not always in conducting a genuine enquiry and reporting on its results.

But are the requirements so transparent? This is a complex question and there is little research which offers guidance, although research on 'the hidden curriculum' may be relevant here. Journals or publishers with an acknowledged political platform (which means they run the risk of being less than purely academic by some criteria) are probably more transparent in broader terms; for example, it would not be wise to submit an anti-feminist article to a feminist journal nor a reactionary manuscript to a left press. However, where the politics are not acknowledged judgments can still be made about what will be seen as suitable and what will not.

Kuhn (1975) has suggested that those who have established reputations (and who are likely to be editors, reviewers or advisors) often have a vested interest in preserving the authority of their work and can suppress fundamental novelties which challenge, or reflect unfavourably on their work (p.5-7). This can lead to a situation where, rather than opening up new developments (and this is significant in feminist terms) many academic publication outlets could be resistant to them, as an effort is made − consciously or unconsciously − to protect those who have 'authority' (see Margrit Eichler, 1981).

The possibility of direct rejection may not even arise, for academics who are seeking publication may deduce that material which conflicts with, or contradicts established authority figures (who may be the editors, reviewers or advisors), will not get published, and while they may disagree with the prevailing orthodoxy, and on good grounds, they may continue to deliver manuscripts which are going to be viewed favourably. By such means can issues be maintained, after evidence which can repudiate them has been accumulated but is unpublished, and sometimes likely to remain unpublished. This can lead to the structural exclusion of those groups whose values and beliefs do not always coincide with the values and beliefs of the gatekeepers. For gatekeepers are in a position to perpetuate their own schemata by exercising sponsorship and patronage towards those who classify the world in ways similar to their own. Women are by no means the only 'outsiders' but they are a significant group and there is considerable evidence which suggests that women's schemata does not at times 'match' with men's.

June Arnold (1976) has commented on this. She has said that some women have known that before they have begun to write 'you had to preprogram your mind to work from male values . . . or you might as well save your pencil for the grocery list' (p.19). But while men are the gatekeepers, such differences can be discounted (see Shirley Ardener, 1975; Dale Spender, 1980; Dorothy Smith, 1978; Virginia Woolf, 1972). This is not necessarily the result of deliberate policy to exclude women (or any other group which does not share the values and beliefs of the gatekeepers) but is the product of closed debate where such groups are not represented and their views, therefore, not heard.

Numerous conventions have evolved which may be unproblematic to those who are the gatekeepers, but which can constitute considerable problems for those who are not. For example, convention favours the publication of results of *successful* experiments, and while this may appear an innocuous practice on the surface, it has numerous implications for women. In my own research on language and sex, for example, I came to the conclusion that the basic assumption behind much of the research was that there was something *wrong* with women's language. One of the predominant research designs was to test the language of women for deficiency and some published articles purported to find what it was that women were doing 'wrong' (Hartman, 1976; Lakoff, 1975; Trudgill, 1975). But very few articles in mainstream academic outlets reported that they had tested women's language for all manner of deficiencies and had *not* found them. (There are however, some feminist articles; see, for example, Kramer *et al.*, 1978, in *Signs*.)

Within such a framework of female deficiency (a framework by no means confined to language research) it becomes very difficult to have findings of 'no difference' reported in the literature, because if the purpose of research is to find where females are deficient, and the deficiency cannot be located, then the experiment can be classified as a failure (rather than as a 'breakthrough' to a reconceptualisation of the problem). And it seems that few failures are reported in the literature, certainly in relation to the social sciences. It is *success* which is favoured among the gatekeepers.

So, while it is perfectly possible that many researchers are finding that there is NO DIFFERENCE between the sexes on many linguistic — or other — items (that is, that their performance can be construed as 'equal'), knowledge of sex 'differences' which frequently portrays women as deficient is still being constructed and disseminated by some academic journals.

One way, then, in which the parameters are constructed is through this disposition to favour so-called successful results. The conceptualisation of the sexes as different — rather than similar or the same — is reinforced and perpetuated through publication, whether this is or is not the most common finding in research; but it is a finding which favours men.

The criteria

The days when we could naively assume that knowledge and truth presented themselves in unadulterated form to scholars who simply and neutrally recorded the phenomena around them are long since past. We have become increasingly aware of the role played by the subjective (partly through feminist efforts) in the construction of knowledge. But I suspect that there is still a level of naivety when it comes to our assumptions about publishing. The criteria which are used to discriminate between what is suitable and what is not, when known, should hardly encourage us to have confidence in the printed word. These criteria frequently reflect the operation of male dominance.

Common sense and some personal experience suggest that not all manuscripts which are submitted receive the same attention. The first decision made by editors confronted with an unsolicited manuscript (commissioned ones are often a very different matter) is whether or not to proceed further, and numerous criteria may be used in the first quick appraisal which can result in a two-line rejection slip or a letter expressing interest. *Form* more often than *content* can be an influential factor, so that considerations such as legibility, accuracy in footnoting and referencing, and so on, are important. 'Carelessness' in other areas, and the *presentation* of material (which includes such things as 'neatness') may become a primary factor in the assessment of scholarly excellence. (There is also the important fact that copy editing, which such careless manuscripts require, is a time-consuming and expensive task.)

But if it passes the first quick assessment stage, and if the editor decides that the topic is interesting and the issue worth pursuing (and in the case of a book manuscript that there is a market for it) then the next item on the agenda is usually to have someone 'vouch' for it. This is where reviewers come in. A lot of reviewing takes place within the academic community and much of it is anonymous. When it is appreciated that there are approximately 2,700 scholarly journals in the USA alone, which receive hundreds more articles than can be included in their pages (Maeroff, 1979) then it can be seen that *space* plays a role in reviewing.

Given the sheer numbers of manuscripts, I think it fair to say that the process is weighted in favour of rejection. (My own experience suggests that reviewers reject far more articles than they accept.) But it is not necessarily space considerations alone that are responsible for this pattern of 'rejecting' behaviour. While many factors may play a contributing role, I suspect that for some there is also an ego-enhancing element in being able to reject the work of one's peers, and in the highly competitive academic world, this should not be overlooked.

But if reviewers are protected by anonymity, writers frequently are not and this has led many writers to claim that the process of selection is far from 'objective' and is biased in favour of those who already have a reputation or have come from a prestigious institution (which could well be a profile of those who are doing the reviewing and who are sponsoring or favouring those in 'their own image')' There has been considerable protest about this in the USA in relation to academic journals and (Maeroff, 1979, p.14)

> there is an increasing interest in a system of anonymous submissions ... to shield the identity of authors from reviewers ... The advocates of this approach maintain that it is more objective because it prevents the reviewers

from favouring the work of better known scholars from the more prestigious universities.

Gene Maeroff goes on to say that among the most ardent proponents of anonymous submissions are younger academics — and women. 'They suspect', he says, 'that they are placed at a disadvantage in competing with more established researchers for the scarce space that is available in journals' (p.C4).

No doubt 'blind refereeing' helps to remove some of the sources of prejudice. Knowing the sex of the writer (apart from her or his place in the pecking order) can be influential in determining whether a piece of work is seen as 'impressive' or 'mediocre' (see Goldberg, 1976). But simply eliminating some of the subjective elements does not necessarily mean that the process becomes 'objective' and that the (elusive) criteria of scholarly excellence can function unimpeded.

Before the reviewers select what is to be published, they themselves are selected and 'subjective' factors can operate here. Reviewing and advising is often a thankless task. Apart from the fact that it is anonymous and even at times secretive (which means that it is not always useful in the public arena) reviewing book-length manuscripts is usually poorly paid, and reviewing articles for academic journals not paid at all. The appointment of reviewers is not open or advertised but usually associated with 'contacts' and 'friends'. This can mean that the range of influence of the editor can extend into the reviewing process itself, for one usually has 'contacts' and 'friends' with whom one 'agrees' on fundamental issues. I am acutely conscious of the significance of the appointment of reviewers. While editing a journal, I have kept my own notes and undertaken my own 'research on research'. On many (if not most) occasions, I can predict whether a reviewer will find an article acceptable and this is not on the basis of conventional criteria of scholarly excellence. Because of the overt political nature of feminism, these predictions are sometimes not difficult to make, and although I would like to tell a different tale, and claim that feminists are completely 'open-minded', I have to state that many feminist reviewers find unacceptable those articles that do not share their own political beliefs. There are few departures from the pattern of rejecting material which is not consistent with one's own viewpoint.

As an editor this constitutes something of a dilemma for me. If I like an article it is not difficult for me to 'choose' two reviewers whom I suspect will also like it, and who will 'justify' my assessment; by the same token, if I do not like it, it is not difficult to 'choose' two reviewers who will not like it either. This hardly seems to be 'objective', or even fair.

No solution can be found by choosing one reviewer who will be favourably disposed towards it, and one who will not, because I can then be left with the deciding vote — or the alternative of choosing yet another reviewer and beginning the process all over again.

I do not want to give this particular facet of the reviewing process undue emphasis. What I want to do is to point out that I (and my 'friends') are aware that this subjective element can and does operate. But instead of being silent about our 'shortcomings' we would prefer to open up the topic for debate. We do not assume that the deficiency lies necessarily in us, but in the belief that there can be an objective process for assessing scholarly excellence. We recognise that we need to 'rethink' the methods by which material is accepted or rejected. This, however, does not seem to have been a significant topic for discussion within the research community as such. Perhaps there has been a 'gentleman's agreement' not to discuss (or disclose) the limitations of the existing system, for I can find few references to the matter in academic literature. In the 1980 series on academic journals in the *Times Higher Education Supplement* this aspect of academic publishing is not discussed and I think this requires explanation.

There is no reason that this problem should be peculiar to feminist journals, and I am assuming that it is only feminists who are prepared to acknowledge the problem, to document the biases which flourish in the selection for publication, and who are trying to find new means of assessment. That there is no such effort being made within mainstream journals also suggests that current practices are not problematic for those who are doing the gatekeeping. If it were, they are in a privileged position to decree it an issue.

Because of the silence which surrounds selection, it is difficult to document the practices and prejudices which occur. But I think it must be accepted that the belief that there is an objective, or even just process which guarantees that the best, the most scholarly, the most enlightening and novel manuscripts are those which find their way to publication, is misguided. What can be said is that we need more research in this area and we need to be aware of present limitations while trying to seek more equitable and justifiable means of dividing the 'rejected' from the 'accepted'.

Male gatekeepers

Most of the data I have used here has been drawn from my own experience and I am mindful of the fact that generalisations made on the basis of one case study have not been encouraged within the academic community. Besides, my experience is not typical; the editors, advisors and reviewers in the academic world are predominantly male.[2] However, rather than seeing this as a reason for *not* making generalisations, I am prepared to use my own entry to what has been previously an area of primarily male privilege as a basis for discussing gatekeeping and for elaborating on the significance of male control of this position.

That there are now feminist publishers, and mainstream publishers who produce feminist journals and books, does mean that there are some outlets for feminist manuscripts which are not monitored by men. But by confining themselves to purely feminist channels, by staying outside the range of influence of the male gatekeepers, feminists may be faced with two dilemmas. First, it is precisely because they are outside male control, and because they do not have to meet male 'standards' that feminist material is often seen to be deficient or lacking in comparison with the male equivalent. That feminist material might not be accepted by men can become evidence that it is not as good as that produced by men. But the second problem is that if feminists do not submit their material to mainstream journals or publishers and seek publication outside feminist channels, then many men and women have good grounds for pleading ignorance when it comes to feminist analysis and insights. Although significant, it is nonetheless insufficient to confine feminist materials to feminist channels, feminists need to enter the mainstream. But as Margrit Eichler (1981) points out, this is where the problem can begin, for men are in control of the mainstream and it seems that 'collectively speaking, our in-roads into mainstream social science have been quite negligible. Overall, social science has been happily able to ignore the work that is being done by feminist scholars' (in press).

It is not just because we need to address non-feminists as well as feminists that feminists need to begin to tackle male dominance of the mainstream, but because we need to conceptualise what is *mainstream* and what is *marginal*. While males are the centre, then feminist analyses and feminist insights are often merely 'tolerated'.

Publishers are not altruistic; with the exception of feminist publishers there are few if any publishers producing feminist periodicals or books because they are committed to the cause. Feminist journals and books are marketed by main-stream publishers because they sell. If they were to cease being profitable, they would cease being published. Whereas a reduction in sales in books about men is likely to be interpre-ted as part of an economic recession, a reduction in sales on books about women could be used as evidence that the 'fashion' has finished, the market has been saturated, and that the scene can revert once more to 'normal'. There is no need to spell out the significance of this.

There was certainly as much, if not more, feminist activity and output during first-wave feminism than has yet been achieved today (see Elizabeth Sarah, 1980) but it 'passed' and it is possible that history could repeat itself. While our gains may appear to be great they may not be as solid nor as enduring as we might like to think. June Arnold (1976) has made a similar observation; in speaking on what it was like before there were contemporary feminist outlets, she has said (p.19) that

If you were very clever and managed to include your voice inside their (male) language *and* get published, you were misreviewed by male papers and your work soon went out of print for economic (political) reasons. The words of earlier feminists were lost because they were the property of male publishers who easily avoided reprinting them.

This can happen again while male-decreed issues constitute the mainstream and males are guarding the gates. We need both a strong feminist base *and* a feminist venture into male territory.

We also need strategies for dismantling male domination of gatekeeping. At the moment, the very structures have been designed to preclude women and their schemata, so that we are often confronted with a vicious circle; for as Eichler (1981 in press) points out, while

mainstream media reject materials that smack even faintly of feminism, nothing will get published within them that challenges their sexism in terms acceptable to them, and consequently, the prevailing scholarly sexism will continue to divert young scholars from doing non-sexist research while reassuring established scholars that there really is no need to change their approach'.

This constitutes an obstacle but it is not one which is impossible to overcome.

Because we recognise that the printed word has an aura of authority, particularly in the academic context, and because we recognise that issues can be formulated and shaped through the process of selecting what gets printed and what does not, we are in a position to use what we know, and to print what has previously not been printed. We can use some of the outlets we have and create new outlets to focus attention on gatekeeping and male control.

If feminist scholars were to document the sex of the editors and advisory boards of journals in their discipline, if within a year they were to itemise the number of articles within a specific mainstream journal that were written about men, by men and for men (and contrast that with the number in which women are theorists or subjects as Sandra Acker (1980) has done for instance) then we would be well prepared — even by male standards — in our arguments about and against male control of this aspect of the construction and distribution of knowledge. To take one example, the *British Education Research Journal* has an all-male editorial board and in the course of one year (1979) published one article by a woman (on primary education) and two articles in which women were co-authors. As there is no shortage of women in the educational field, what were the factors operating to exclude women? And how can this inequality be justified? If the justification were in terms of academic excellence then the material selected should be subjected to closer scrutiny and some attempt made to examine that which was rejected. This could be done by making an appeal — perhaps in the pages of the *British Education Research Journal* — for those who were rejected to come forward, and help provide the data for research on male control of these channels.

In silence, many current practices are protected, and it is only by breaking that silence that male control can be exposed. Speaking out on a topic that has been shrouded in silence has become a characteristic of feminist research and once more we need to make problematic what has previously been taken too much for granted. We need to do some research on research at the level of publication.

Already some efforts are being made in this area. Margrit Eichler, for example, has published a shortened version of an article that was rejected by mainstream journals, and she has published an appendix with it which includes the reviewers' reports and rejections. She ends her appendix with the following statement (Eichler, 1981):

> I suggest that we research the history of feminist scholarship by making public the experience of feminist scholars in producing and publishing non-sexist materials in a sexist scholarly environment. This should provide us with a data set from which to attack the continuing sexist exclusion of feminist thought. This means that all of us will have to go through our private closets to sort out what in our experience qualifies as sexist

discrimination. . . . Hopefully, such effort will enable us to expose sexist gatekeeping as just that. While such exposure will not guarantee that the practice will cease, it will certainly put us in a better position to argue for the need to revise current gatekeeping criteria. And that, at least, would mean a small foot in the door.

When such material appears in print, it is *quotable*, it beomes reportable if not reputable by male standards. It enjoys the benefits of legitimation that accompany the printed word; we know this and should use it.

I think this should be a fundamental aspect of 'doing feminist research', for unless we are equally represented among the gatekeepers and unless our values and concerns are seen to be as valid as those of men, much of our current research may never reach the reported stage, and much of our reported research may 'disappear' in the future. Part of research is publication, and changing the power configurations in the publishing process should be a priority item on the feminist research agenda.

Notes

1   There are exceptions — particularly if the 'private communication' is with an eminent scholar in which case the status of the writer can be enhanced by virtue of being in receipt of a 'private communication' from such an eminent source.

2   Of all the many academic journals published by Pergamon Press, for instance, there are only two women editors — myself and the editor of a nursing journal. There is no reason for suspecting that this pattern is atypical.

References

Acker, Sandra (1980), 'Feminist perspectives on the British Sociology of Education', paper presented at British Sociological Association Annual Conference, Lancaster, 8 April.

Ardener, Shirley (ed.) (1975), *Perceiving Women*, Malaby, London.

Arnold, June (1976), 'Feminist Presses and Feminist Politics', *Quest: a Feminist Quarterly*, vol. III, no. 1, pp.18–26.

Buchan, Lou (1980), 'Private communication' on research for book,

Unpublished Heritage: the Politics of Selection, forthcoming from Pergamon Press, Oxford.

Eichler, Margrit (1981); (in press), 'Power, dependency, love and the sexual division of labour: a critique of the decision-making approach to family power and an alternative approach with an appendix: On washing my dirty linen in public', *Women's Studies International Quarterly*, vol. IV, no. 2.

Goldberg, Philip (1976), 'Are women prejudiced against women' in Judith Stacey *et al.* (eds), *And Jill Came Tumbling After: Sexism in American Education*, Dell, New York, pp.37–42.

Hartman, Maryann (1976), 'A descriptive study of the language of men and women born in Maine around 1900 as it reflects the Lakoff hypothesis in "Language and Women's [sic] Place"' in I. Dubois and B. Crouch (eds), *The Sociology of the Language of American Women*, Pise Papers IV, Trinity University, San Antonio, Texas, pp.81–90.

Kramer, Cheris, Thorne, Barrie, and Henley, Nancy, (1978), 'Perspectives on Language and Communication', *Signs: Journal of Women in Culture and Society*, vol. III, no. 3, pp.638–51.

Kuhn, Thomas (1975), *The Structure of Scientific Revolutions* (2nd edn.), University of Chicago Press.

Lakoff, Robin (1975), *Language and Woman's Place*, Harper & Row, New York.

Maeroff, Gene I. (1979), 'Journals' problem: what to publish?', *New York Times*, 14 August, pp.C1 and C4.

Sarah, Elizabeth (1980), paper on first wave feminism given at the Women's Research and Resources Centre Conference, 'The Women's Liberation Movement and Men', London, 23 March.

Smith, Dorothy (1978), 'A Peculiar Eclipsing: Women's Exclusion from Man's Culture', *Women's Studies International Quarterly*, vol. I, no. 4. pp.281–96.

Spender, Dale (1980), 'A Feminist Critique of Education', forthcoming article in the *Times Higher Education Supplement*.

Spender, Dale (ed.) (1981), *Men's Studies Modified: The Impact of Feminism on the Academic Disciplines*, Pergamon Press, Oxford.

Trudgill, Peter (1975), 'Sex, Covert Prestige and Linguistic Change in the Urban British English of Norwich' in Barrie Thorne and Nancy Henley (eds), *Language and Sex: Difference and Dominance*, Newbury House, Mass. pp.88–104.

Woolf, Virginia (1972), 'Women and Fiction', first published in *The Forum* March 1928, Reprinted in Leonard Woolf, (ed.), *Collected Essays: Virginia Woolf*, vol. II, Chatto & Windus, London, pp.141–8.

Index

203